The TRUTH

HAY HOUSE TITLES OF RELATED INTEREST

Books

BodyChange™: *The 21-Day Fitness Program for Changing Your Body . . . and Changing Your Life!*
by Montel Williams and Wini Linguvic

Every Move You Make: *Bodymind Exercises to Transform Your Life,* by Nikki Winston

Flex Ability: *A Story of Strength and Survival,* by Flex Wheeler, with Cindy Pearlman

I'm Still Hungry: *Finding Myself Through Thick and Thin,* by Carnie Wilson, with Cindy Pearlman

Shape® Magazine's Shape Your Life: *4 Weeks to a Better Body—and a Better Life,*
by Barbara Harris, editor-in-chief, *Shape* magazine, with Angela Hynes

The TOPS Way to Weight Loss: *Beyond Calories and Exercise,* by Howard Rankin, Ph.D.

Ultimate Pilates, by Dreas Reyneke

Yoga Pure and Simple, by Kisen

The Yo-Yo Diet Syndrome: *How to Heal and Stabilize Your Appetite and Weight,*
by Doreen Virtue, Ph.D.

Card Decks

8 Minutes in the Morning® Kit: *A Simple Way to Shed Up to
2 Pounds a Week Guaranteed,* by Jorge Cruise

I Can Do It® Cards: *Affirmations for Health,* by Louise L. Hay

OM Yoga in a Box, by Cyndi Lee

All of the above are available at your local bookstore, or may be ordered
by visiting any of the following Hay House Websites: Hay House USA: **www.hayhouse.com;**
Hay House Australia: **www.hayhouse.com.au;** Hay House U.K.: **www.hayhouse.co.uk;**
or Hay House South Africa: **orders@psdprom.co.za**

The TRUTH

The *Only* Fitness Book You'll Ever Need

FRANK SEPE

HAY HOUSE

HAY HOUSE, INC.
Carlsbad, California
London • Sydney • Johannesburg
Vancouver • Hong Kong

Copyright © 2003 by Frank Sepe

Published and distributed in the United States by: Hay House, Inc., P.O. Box 5100, Carlsbad, CA 92018-5100 • *Phone:* (760) 431-7695 or (800) 654-5126 • *Fax:* (760) 431-6948 or (800) 650-5115 • www.hayhouse.com • **Published and distributed in Australia by:** Hay House Australia, Ltd., 18/36 Ralph St., Alexandria NSW 2015 • *Phone:* 612-9669-4299 • *Fax:* 612-9669-4144 • www.hayhouse.com.au • **Published and Distributed in the United Kingdom by:** Hay House UK, Ltd. • Unit 202, Canalot Studios • 222 Kensal Rd., London W10 5BN • *Phone:* 44-20-8962-1230 • *Fax:* 44-20-8962-1239 • www.hayhouse.co.uk • **Published and Distributed in the Republic of South Africa by:** Hay House SA (Pty), Ltd., P.O. Box 990, Witkoppen 2068 • *Phone/Fax:* 2711-7012233 • orders@psdprom.co.za • **Distributed in Canada by:** Raincoast • 9050 Shaughnessy St., Vancouver, B.C. V6P 6E5 • *Phone:* (604) 323-7100 • *Fax:* (604) 323-2600

Editorial supervision: Jill Kramer
Book design: Summer McStravick
Fitness photography: Myrna Suarez/TwinBPhotography.com
Photos of Frank Sepe: Mike Ruiz

All rights reserved. No part of this book may be reproduced by any mechanical, photographic, or electronic process, or in the form of a phonographic recording; nor may it be stored in a retrieval system, transmitted, or otherwise be copied for public or private use—other than for "fair use" as brief quotations embodied in articles and reviews without prior written permission of the publisher.

The author of this book does not dispense medical advice or prescribe the use of any technique as a form of treatment for physical or medical problems without the advice of a physician, either directly or indirectly. The intent of the author is only to offer information of a general nature to help you in your quest for emotional and spiritual well-being. In the event you use any of the information in this book for yourself, which is your constitutional right, the author and the publisher assume no responsibility for your actions.

Library of Congress Cataloging-in-Publication Data

Sepe, Frank, 1971-
  The truth : the only fitness book you'll ever need / Frank Sepe.
    p. cm.
  ISBN 1-4019-0168-9 (hardcover) — ISBN 1-4019-0179-4 (tradepaper) 1. Physical fitness. 2. Exercise. 3. Nutrition. I. Title.
  GV481.S37 2003
  613.7'1—dc21
                          2003005886

Hardcover ISBN 1-4019-0168-9
Tradepaper ISBN 1-4019-0179-4

06 05 04 03   4 3 2 1
1st printing, October 2003

Printed in the United States of America

In loving memory of Alice Kohlhepp.

*This book is also dedicated to my
mother and father, and my wife, Lisa.*

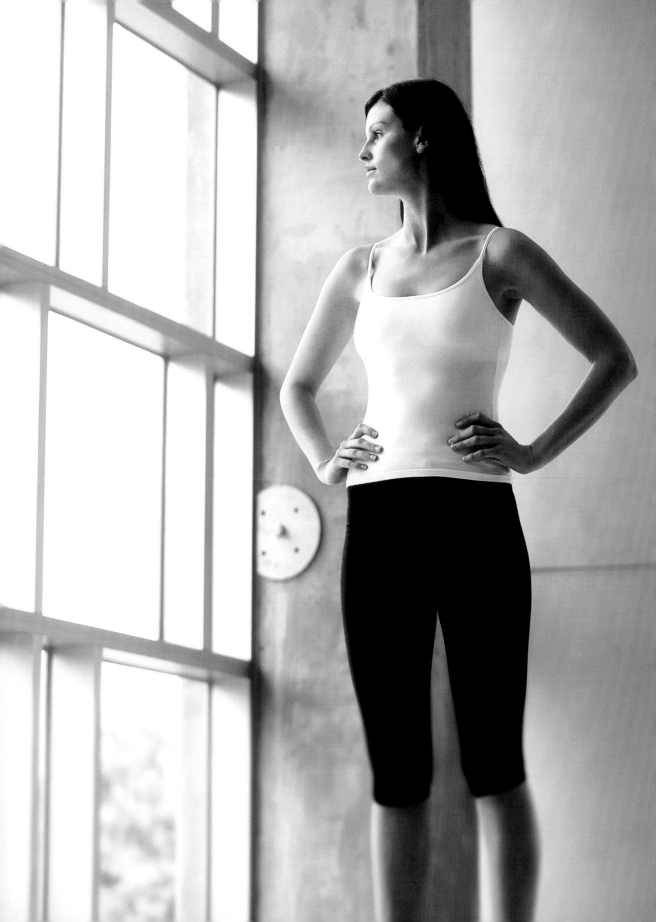

Contents

(**Author's Note:** Always consult your physician or other health-care provider before beginning any exercise, nutritional, or weight-loss program, especially if you suffer from a bad back, heart disease, or other medical problem or condition. If you're going to engage in weight-training exercise, I recommend that you consult with a licensed fitness trainer or expert.)

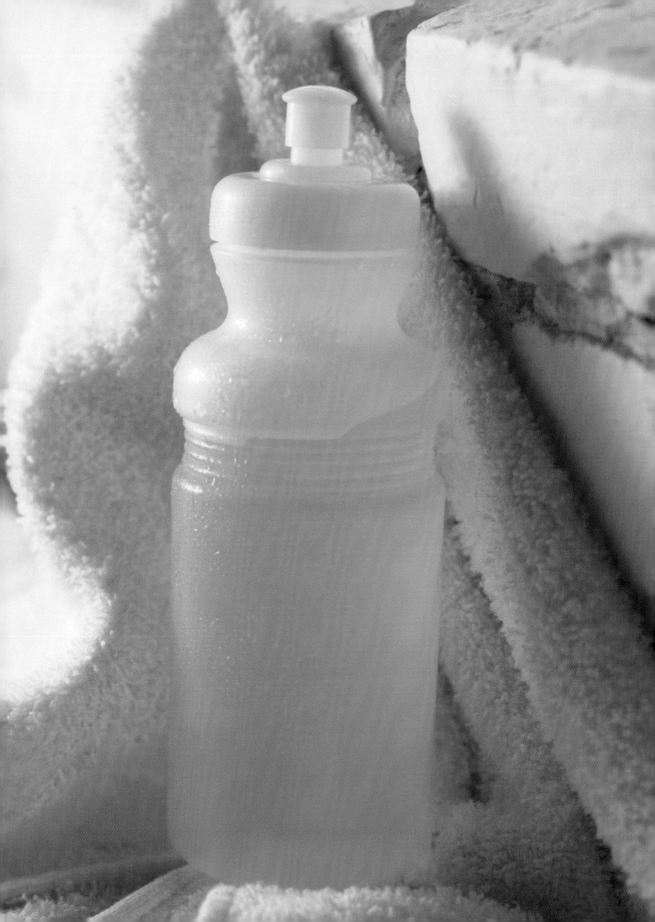

Acknowledgments

A person's wealth should never be measured in dollars and cents, but by his or her friends and family. Therefore, I consider myself one of the richest people on Earth. I've been blessed with a wonderful and loving family—my mom, Mary; and my dad, Thomas, have always put the love of their family first. I don't have the words to thank them enough for the constant unconditional love and support they've shown me my entire life. I'm truly blessed and extremely fortunate to have these two remarkable people in my life.

They say that behind every good man is a good woman—my wife, Lisa, is that woman. She's made every day I spend on this planet better than the last, and I'd like to thank her for showing me that sometimes there is indeed a light at the end of the tunnel. I love you.

Special thanks to:

Reid Tracy and Danny Levin from Hay House for being so supportive and enthusiastic about this project. I thank you both from the bottom of my heart for giving me the opportunity to make a positive difference in so many people's lives.

Steve Weinberger—thank you for being such a great friend over the years. You've been like a brother to me, and your advice and teachings have played a huge role in the success I've achieved thus far. I have the utmost respect and admiration for you as a person, and I'm honored to call you my friend.

Robert Kennedy—it was your publication, *MuscleMag International,* that started it all for me. Thank you for giving me the opportunity to appear in all of your magazines for the past decade. It's because of you that I was able to showcase my talent as a writer, and I can now call myself a published author. It's very rare to remain friends with someone for so long in this industry, but you aren't the average person. I can't thank you enough for your advice, wisdom, and friendship. You are, without a doubt, one of a kind.

The Sepe family—I want to thank all of you for your love and encouragement. I appreciate it a great deal. Thank you Tommy, Susan, Laci, Robin, Uncle Joe, Aunt Cathy, Diane Sepe, Richard Pelcher, and Isabelle and Matthew Pelcher.

John Edward—sometimes we meet people who make an immediate impact on our lives, and you are indeed that person for me. I want to thank you for your priceless advice, friendship, and sense of humor. It's nice to know that there are still some very real and sincere people out there. Thanks.

Bev Francis, Jim Manion, Charlie Chiaverini, Theresa Hartle—thank you all for looking out for me over the years. I appreciate everything you've done for me.

Kerrie Lee Brown—thank you for giving me the opportunity to write my first feature article in *American Health & Fitness.* You've been a great friend and ally in this business. May you and Craig have many, many years of happiness, and may your magazine continue to prosper.

Special thanks also go out to all of the talented individuals who worked so hard on this book:

Cindy Pearlman—thank you for all of your contributions to *The TRUTH.* You've done a superb job whipping this book into shape. It's been a wonderful and fun experience working with you, and I hope I have the privilege of working with you again. Thanks.

Richard Perez Feria—thank you for helping me achieve a personal goal of mine. I want to thank you for your creative vision and for being a solid friend. Mike Ruiz, Myrna Suarez, and Sean Kahlil—thanks for your beautiful photos. Bill Henning; Mary Wiswall; Fred Bimbler; George Slowik, Jr.; and the Gates sisters, Kathleen, Linda, and Susan—thank you for all of your effort and contribution to this book. I appreciate it a great deal.

Larry Pepe—we've been friends for 13 years. Who would have thought back then that we'd be here now educating the world on fitness? I want to thank you for contributing to and helping to develop The TRUTH program into what it has become today. Your expertise and practical knowledge in the fields of psychology, motivation, and nutrition have been invaluable. You have my endorsement now and in the future as one of the most knowledgeable mental and physical teachers someone can have access to. You're definitely an asset to anyone who seeks help in bettering themselves. I look forward to a lifetime of friendship and working together. Thank you.

Thanks to all of my friends at my second home, Bev Francis's Gold's Gym in Syosset, New York.

To Richard Jankura—you've proven to be a great friend, someone I can rely on through thick and thin. Your enthusiasm and positive attitude toward this project and me have definitely helped me get through some rough times. Thank you for being a true friend.

To MET-Rx—it has been my honor and privilege to be associated with such a great company. MET-Rx products have played a huge role in the development of my physique and in my everyday eating plan. I look forward to continue working with MET-Rx in the future.

Dr. Perry Frankel—thanks for looking after me all of these years. You make it posible for me to maintain my level of fitness. Your sincere concern and knowledge has kept me on the road to good health. I am blessed to have you as a doctor and a friend.

Thomas Marinelli—thanks for your support and friendship for the past decade. It has meant a lot to me.

Ralph Potente—thanks for your support and friendship.

Finally, to Steve McGrath—thanks for sticking to the program. Your dedication and effort not only made a difference in your life, but in mine as well.

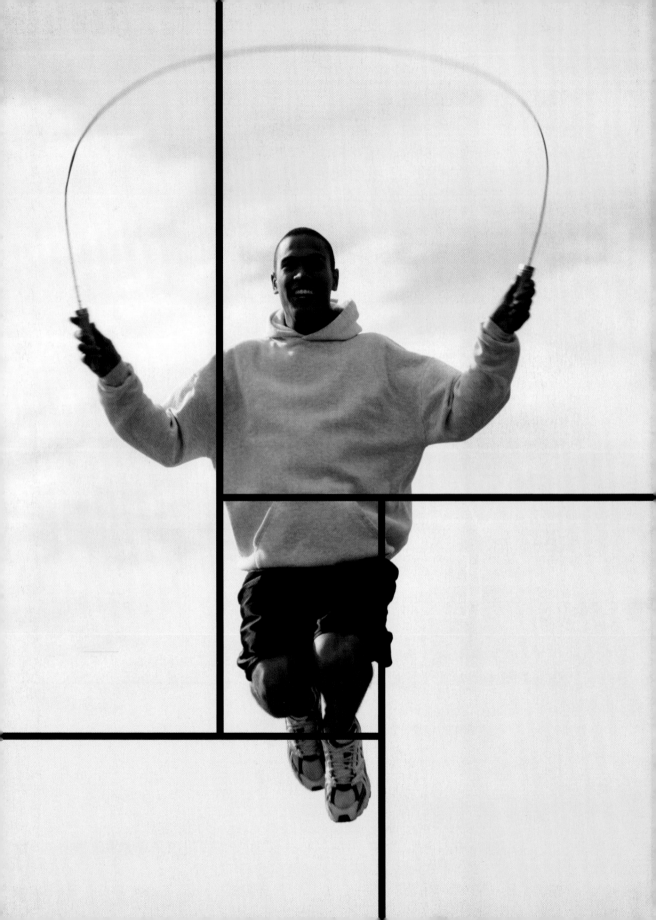

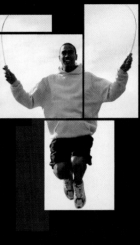

TIME TO TELL THE TRUTH

I hold this *one* truth to be self-evident: Not all diets and workout programs are created equal.

Okay, so I messed with one of the most famous lines from our forefathers, men who flexed their might and not their biceps. But, hey, if we were busy working the fields and eating wild boar again, then none of us would have to work at having the perfect body (or even getting a tan for that matter). Unfortunately, it's the new millennium—where, despite all the stress out there, the most physically strenuous thing most people do during the day is lift their cell phone to their ears, press a cup of coffee to their lips, or strengthen their index fingers while surfing the Internet.

Just by picking up this book, which weighs about a pound, you're starting to do some toning work already. Congratulations! Speaking of what you're reading, I decided to write a fitness book with a twist, and I vow it will be the last fitness book that you'll ever have to buy.

Those are bold words, but I stand behind them because I'm armed with The TRUTH. From this moment on, there will be no more lies when it comes to getting the body you want. I promise not to offer some fad diet or quick fix that promises to get you pumped up with false hope. I know it's confusing because there's so much diet and health info out there, but my program offers solid advice and a workable plan to achieve the body that maybe you've only seen in your dreams.

Believe me, I wish I could just give you some trendy, short-term miracle that would make you say, "This Frank guy is amazing! He claims I can eat chocolate cake, work out only once a week, and get the body of Arnold Schwarzenegger." Yeah, I've read about those plans, too. A few of them have raised my heart rate . . . and not in a good way. Even *I* can't believe what many infomercials, fitness magazines, gyms, and trainers are promising. I'm even more upset by all those ads for diet pills, supplement powders and shakes, and useless home-gym equipment. They might feel good, but vibrating ab stimulators are unsafe and useless. Magic potions only work in cartoons, and some of those diet drugs out there are downright dangerous and even deadly.

This book is not a quick fix—it's a lifestyle. It's about making a physical *and* mental change to get to the true you, or the best you possible.

I know you want to believe that the easy way is the best way, because most of us have been at a point in our lives where we'd do just about anything to have the perfect body. Believe me, I've been there.

Please, let me introduce myself: I'm Frank Sepe, and I used to have a body that made me want to cry. By the time I was 13 years old, I dreaded going to school because the other kids tormented me. The problem was that I was almost 5'9" and maybe 120 pounds, which wasn't a good thing at this sensitive time in a boy's life. (These days, I'm 6'2" and 235 pounds.)

Here's a sample of what the other kids would call me: "beanpole," "bird legs," and "chicken neck." I saved my personal favorite for last, which I'll use in a helpful sentence: "Hey, Frankenstein! Where are the bolts in your neck?"

That was life for the son of a New York City police detective, a kid who was trying to enjoy his otherwise normal childhood in Rosedale, Queens. I had loving parents, an older brother, and a younger sister, and I never let them see how upset I was—but the truth was that the constant taunting really bothered me. My mom wasn't exactly thrilled when I began getting into dozens of fights. And my new tough-guy persona really didn't do anything except get me some deten-tion and make my detractors even more determined to call me names. It got to the point where the names upset me more than being skinny did, yet I was determined to build my body—using the logic of a teenager.

One night, I decided that I was going to eat everything my stomach could hold. I reasoned that this way, I'd naturally gain weight. "I'm going to eat until people stop calling me names," I swore, digging into a gallon of chocolate ice cream. I also ate a pound of bologna, figuring that I would gain an actual pound. Well, let's just say that ice cream and bologna don't mix well. After spending an hour in the kitchen trying to fatten myself up, I was on the verge of needing a huge bottle of Pepto-Bismol, so I decided to take a break. That's when I heard a banging noise in the basement. Hoping that it wasn't a burglar, I decided to check it out, and that's when I saw something that would change my life forever.

My father was the one making all the racket. "I'm bench-pressing," he grunted, while lift-ing what seemed to be 1,000 pounds (it was really about 300). When he finished his set and put the weight back on the rack, it made this loud clanking noise that sounded like someone banging a gong in victory. I remained frozen in that same spot at the top of the stairs for a good hour, just watching my dad, and my eyes bugged out as he kept adding weights. Now, my dad was a very muscular guy, but he needed that strength because he was a cop. Of course I'd seen his biceps bursting from his T-shirts, but I never thought about how he got so brawny.

Then it dawned on me: *If Dad made his muscles, then maybe I can build up some of those babies, too.* Later that night, my stomach in agony from all that food, my mind raced while I tried to go to sleep. All I could think was, *I'll start working out and get big, and nobody will ever mess with me again.*

Ever the super-sleuth, I hid on those basement stairs for a week and secretly wrote down everything my dad was doing. Thus, my first training routine was born. There was a tiny glitch, however—the basement was off-limits to me and dubbed "a private spot" for my dad and older brother to train. Mom, who was always worrying about me, said, "Frank, you're way too young to lift weights." I couldn't blame her for her concern, but I defied her anyway. I did what any nor-mal 13-year-old would do under the circumstances—I snuck into the basement to work out when nobody was home. Luckily, my family went out quite a lot, so for three months, I got to train almost every single day . . . and then I got caught. "Frank, we told you to stay the heck out of the base-ment," Mom said. "Oh, I'll never go down there again," I swore, counting the moments until she and Dad pulled out of the driveway. Two seconds later, my hands were wrapped around those cold steel barbells.

The second time I was nailed, my exasperated parents discussed the situation, and my dad finally said, "Let him stay down there. At least he's not annoying any of us up in the regular part of the house." With that kind of go-ahead, I was psyched. I began to follow Dad's workout routine, training for two hours a day, six days a week.

Lo and behold, old Frankenstein began to get a little broader, but I was still a far cry from being an official "big guy." Mentally, it was a different story, because I was feeling much stronger on that front. I *knew* I wasn't going to let anyone bring me down anymore, and that's what got me through training during the hot air-conditioner-free days of summer and the heatless nights of winter. Then came the fateful night when my dad wandered down the basement steps to check on me and was actually impressed. "Let me give you some tips," he said.

That Christmas, I didn't get a radio-controlled car from my father—instead, I got a 45-pound plate and an incline bench. Pop was obviously proud, to the point that he videotaped my entire workout so that he could give me pointers on how to improve. (Who would have guessed that that tape would air on national television ten years later?) The moral of the story is: It's a good thing my parents let me use that basement, which I practically lived in from ages 13 to 17. Needless to say, my body changed drastically. I bulked up to 215 pounds of pure muscle. The perks were amazing . . . especially when the girls at school checked me out while the guys asked for workout tips. That wasn't half bad for a guy who had the most basic gym equipment and little knowledge of proper nutrition. As for those kids who used to beat me up—well, now they avoided me at all costs. Yes, life was looking up.

WHEN I WAS 17, I started to train at a local gym. Just joining it was sort of a funny experience because Joe, the guy behind the desk, took one look at me and asked, "Are you a policeman or a fireman? We can give you the rate for civil-service workers."

It seems that in those days, the only toned guys in town were cops and firemen, not 17-year-olds. When I told Joe how old I was, he dropped his pen and said, "Hang on—you're just a kid? How did you get so big?" A second later, he invited a group of bodybuilders to the front counter and asked, "How old do you think this guy is?"

A rather large man named Charlie looked me up and down and barked, "Who cares? He has no legs."

Ouch! And this came from a guy with no neck. This hurt because it was the first time in years that I'd been confronted by a negative remark about my physique. "Hey, I might have no legs now, but I just joined. What's *your* excuse?" Charlie looked at me with a shocked expression. Before I could run out of there, I added, "One day you'll be asking me how I got my legs so big."

Charlie smiled and said, "Score one for the kid," chuckling as he walked away.

Apparently, all my bravado also made a big impression on Joe. Yep, it turns out that he wasn't just some counter guy after all—he was also a national weightlifting champion with numerous records. He said, "Kid, I like you, and I'm going to train you myself." From that day on, Joe kept an eye on me and told me when I was doing something wrong. Let's put it this way: He wasn't a very quiet person. But after the first day at his gym, I came home with an amazing new training routine that taught me about equipment I'd utilize years later when I discovered The TRUTH.

Let's not get too ahead of ourselves just yet, though. I graduated from high school and began to take college classes at Nassau Community College. I studied criminal justice (like father, like son) for two years, and gathered enough units for an associate degree. However, the highlight of my day wasn't exactly my classes—it was going to the gym, where I made it my business to train with different partners. I figured that if I could pick up one tip or training secret from each person, then I'd be ahead of the game. And being a competitive type of guy, I excelled at all the new moves much faster than the other people in the gym.

Joe noticed that I was in über-workout mode one day, so he decided to give me a little test. "Work out with me, Frank," he said, knowing that he was much stronger than I was, and eventually I'd either throw up or throw in the towel. After 30 sets of 20 squats, I could barely stand, but I didn't quit. "You have the heart of a champion, kid," he said, and that was one of the nicest things I ever heard in my life.

When I was 19, I met my friend Larry Pepe in the most normal way. We started talking at the gym about bodybuilding, figuring that we had a lot in common despite the fact that Larry was nine years older than I was and was preparing for a natural bodybuilding contest. "I need someone to train with me," he said, and I took him up on his offer. We trained together seven days a week, each pushing the other one to new places. Larry also introduced me to the concept of nutrition, which was a whole new world for a kid who figured that hot dogs were a major food group.

"What's an eating plan?" I asked, as I polished off a carb-loaded blueberry muffin from Dunkin' Donuts. (Why are these places always around the corner from gyms, I ask you?)

At the time, I was eating everything I could to pack weight on. Larry told me that I had to be careful about what I ate, which included limiting my sodium and carbs. A few weeks later, I was training, eating, and best of all, *looking* like a bodybuilder. For the first time in my life—

despite all of my previous years of working out—I actually had definition and separation in my muscles. I had a six-pack stomach back in the days when that term was reserved for the amount of beer some of my friends downed when they partied on the weekends. I didn't have time for drinking anything except water because I spent my weekends at the gym. Every time I looked in the mirror, I couldn't help but think, *Wow! I'm never eating fried chicken again.* I even tried to pass some of my new know-how on to others, starting a small personal-training program on the side to earn extra cash for school. Even as a young guy, I loved helping people get what they wanted out of their bodies. When I saw someone who had been struggling to reach a goal actually attain it, it was like I'd done it myself.

By the time I was 21, I was done with college and decided to give professional bodybuilding a shot. I found myself in Manhattan when something amazing happened. A man approached me and said, "I'm a modeling scout, and if you're interested in making some really great money, you should give me a call." Now, this was the kind of dough I needed in my life! Before I knew it, I had a legitimate reason for working out: It paid the bills! My first real job was for a fashion magazine called *U Interview,* and I guess my look went over big, because soon I was booking job after job. I shot everything—greeting cards, catalogs, magazines—you name it. Around this time, I also made a conscious decision to change my training program at the gym. I didn't need to build mass, but to stay sinewy and strong.

Obviously, this was the right way to pursue modeling, because I soon got a call from my agent saying that Joan Rivers was looking for a bodybuilder to star in a TV promo for her talk show. It wasn't a done deal, so I had to audition. This was interesting in and of itself, because soon I was in a room with professional bodybuilders, exotic dancers, and just about every beefy model from the greater New York area and Canada, too. In the waiting room, I kept hearing, "You're Frank Sepe, right?" Hold on just a second: How did these people even know my name? It didn't dawn on me that I was actually building up a good reputation as a model along with my muscles.

By the way, I got the job with Joan, although you might not remember me. At the time, she was more preoccupied with her dog, Spike. Ignored in favor of a little furball with sharp teeth . . . oh well, that's showbiz.

I wasn't completely satisfied with modeling. Deep down, I still wanted to give bodybuilding a shot, so I started some serious training to compete in the Eastern States Bodybuilding Championships. I managed to get in great shape at 240 pounds (not bad for a 22-year-old), and I won the heavyweight class and the "Most Muscular" awards.

Afterwards, I chose to return to modeling and yes, I booked the centerfold for *Playgirl.* What?

Did you think it would take much longer before we got to the good stuff? I have to be honest, though—my girlfriend at the time didn't exactly appreciate all this exposure, but I told her, "Honey, people are just admiring my physique. I worked really hard to get my body in this shape." Even now, people ask me if I regret posing for *Playgirl*. Of course everyone has regrets, but that's not one of mine. I was happy with the photos and the response I got from many devoted fans. Yep, I now had fans.

I also believe that taking this risk helped me get my name out there to an even greater degree, which is why I also nabbed a role in the Al Pacino film *Carlito's Way*. Life was good, and it got even better when I took another six months off to prepare for the 1995 Metropolitan Body-building Championships, which I won. Now, things were really jumping because ESPN wanted me to shoot a series of segments for a new fitness show. The only downside was that I had to quit training people on the side, despite the fact that by now I was one of the most sought-after personal trainers in my area.

One of the reasons I had to let my clients go was because I knew that I needed to head west to legendary Venice Beach, California, to see where all this fitness work would take me. I worried that I wouldn't go far with only $500 in my pocket and an invitation from my old friend Larry Pepe to stay in his house. But as soon as I touched down in Los Angeles, I found my way to the famous Gold's Gym in Venice where, coincidentally, there were three photo sessions going on at the same time.

As I was training, one of the photographers approached me and said, "I'm not sure if you've ever heard this before, but you should be a model." I laughed and did a few shots with him. A few hours later, the other photographers came by, and I booked five days' worth of shoots with some of bodybuilding's top shutterbugs.

A few weeks later, I decided that the L.A. lifestyle wasn't for me, so I returned home with more than just some happy memories and a tan. Some of the fitness magazines I posed for started to hit the newsstands, and I'll never forget the day when I saw my mug on the cover of *MuscleMag International,* one of bodybuilding's premier magazines. This was a magazine that I couldn't wait to read every single month—I'd even drive to Manhattan to get one because it arrived a week later where I lived. Arnold and Sly had been on the cover of this magazine I'd loved from the time I was 13, and now I was smiling out from that same spot. It was one of the most satisfying moments of my entire life.

In the next few months, I was in almost every fitness magazine on the stands, and my face was seen daily on ESPN's bodybuilding shows. All the exposure paid off in the form of endorsement contracts for companies such as MET-Rx. Soon I was making appearances, doing seminars, and shooting commercials for one of the largest sports-nutrition companies in the world. My face was also going mainstream because *Billboard* magazine shot me for an ad and then the TV series *Hard Copy* shot a segment on me, dubbing me "the most photographed bodybuilder in the world." It was great exposure, made better by the fact that I got my mom and dad on the show. My mother was suddenly signing autographs at the grocery store, which made me one happy camper.

My new brush with fame wasn't enough, though. I set my sights on the North American Body-building Championship, which would pit me against some of the best athletes from the U.S., Mexico, and Canada. Just like when I was a kid, I heard the vicious backstage backbiting the minute I got to the competition. "How long will the young pretty boy last?" one bodybuilder asked with a smirk. "Oh, that Sepe will get crushed. I doubt he'll even make the top 15," said another champion who shall remain nameless. I was the youngest (24), but biggest (260 pounds) competitor in the show and placed fifth.

I didn't have time to think about whether this was good or bad. As I walked out of the venue with my mother and brother, I felt a stabbing pain in my stomach. The pain was so bad that it immediately sent me to my knees, and I ended up on the pavement writhing in pain. That's when the strangest thing happened—my abdominal muscles started protruding out by about two inches. I had to push them back in place with my hands, which caused a pain so excruciating that I almost passed out. A doctor was rushed to the scene, who told my frantic family, "Frank is severely dehydrated, but I can help him."

It's an old story: Sometimes the expectations and the pressure to win becomes so great that we do foolish and dangerous things to try to achieve a goal. That's another reason why I've written this book. *I don't want you to do anything stupid or medically dangerous in the name of losing weight or getting in shape.* Believe me when I say that it's simply not worth it. You can lose big trying to "win at all costs." I've done some things that I'm not proud of in the name of looking my best for a show, but I made a pact with myself after that day on the pavement that I would never sacrifice my health again.

I also decided that this was a major wake-up call. It was time to stop competing and putting my health on the line. I knew I had to redirect my energy into more positive pursuits, and I had an idea that I could take all the years, all the training, and all the know-how, and put it to good use for myself and for other people out there.

"Frank, are you nuts?" bodybuilding friends asked me. "You can win this thing next year. All the magazines are saying that you're the next champ."

"I can't win anything if I'm dead," I told them.

OVER THE NEXT YEAR, I revamped my training and nutritional plan and dropped 50 pounds in five months. Let me just say that it wasn't easy, in case you're about to ask, "How did you do it? I want your diet plan." I trained hard to lose that weight, and mentally I also had to adjust to having a much lighter body weight. My plan worked, because I wasn't just losing the pounds, I was becoming firmer and more defined as I went down on the scale. During this time, I was absolutely flooded with modeling work and appeared on more than 50 national and international magazine covers. Hmm, I guess there was something to this new plan I was inventing, because it truly worked.

Apparently my new form really appealed to the ladies because I was asked to become a romance-novel cover boy and shot more than three dozen book covers for several different companies. It didn't hurt that at the time I was also chosen as one of *Playgirl's* "100 Best Centerfolds of All Time."

The work was fun, and the money was great, but I needed something even more satisfying in my life. That's why I went back to personal training. More than anything, I wanted to help other people achieve fitness goals that seemed impossible. There was nothing I liked better than an initial consultation with a person who would say, "Frank, I've failed my entire life when it comes to getting my body in shape. I know you probably can't really help me either, but I just had to give it a shot." Not help them? Excuse me? The 13-year-old weakling who still lurks deep down inside of me just loved that kind of challenge.

Knowing that I didn't just want to help people from the New York area, I called Bob Kennedy of *MuscleMag International* and asked him if I could write a monthly question-and-answer column. He agreed to let me do it—and hundreds of letters poured in every single week, asking for my advice on everything from toning to skin care to sex (!). I was also asked to write columns for *American Health & Fitness,* a publication for average guys who weren't necessarily into bodybuilding. *Hollywood Shape* magazine also named me as one of New York's top personal trainers. I think my mail carrier nearly got a hernia from all the letters I received after I became a fitness consultant for many TV shows and women's magazines, not to mention sports stars and celebs.

It dawned on me that what I was doing now was much better than competing because instead of building my own body, I was building the self-esteem of other people. Yet in the middle of the night, a few scary thoughts would go through my mind, such as, *Who am I to be giving advice? Do I know enough about health?* So I became almost obsessed with learning as much as possible about different dietary and training techniques. I found that I liked different parts of each of these methods, but none of them appealed to me as a balanced, successful, inspirational program.

How could I tell people the truth about nutrition and fitness? I wasn't even 30 years old, yet I knew that I'd have to put my own program together based on my life experience and the feedback of my clients, who told me such things as, "Thank you for helping me achieve my goal. Now I have the body of my dreams. I never could have done this without your plan."

These are people like you and me who have tried just about every program out there. I knew that my program would be based on a simple fact: The truth is . . . The TRUTH actually works. If you give 100 percent, you'll achieve your goal. If you don't, then you'll fail.

Hey, sometimes The TRUTH hurts, but I have to be honest.

So what is The TRUTH? It's both a diet program and a workout regime. And, as I said before, it's not a quick fix. It isn't easy, but it *is* ultimately worth it. What I'm going to give you in this book is a lifetime plan that's realistic for anyone at any fitness level. We'll exercise together, but just as important, I'll give you a diet plan that really works. Forget this zero-carb business—sure, you'll lose weight, but you'll also lose your sanity. I mean, every once in a while I want to eat a doughnut or a slice of pizza. Does that make me a failure? No, it makes me human.

I'll tell you how to follow my exact diet, which will help you lose weight while still allowing for the occasional indulgence. Even better is that when we get to the exercise part of book, it will be as if I'm your own personal trainer who has come over for a daily workout session, filled with enough instruction, information, and motivation to get you closer to your goals.

This book is divided into three sections. Part I outlines why you need to discover The TRUTH, while Parts II and III give you the actual plan, including detailed exercise instruction to tone up and progress from a beginner's level to an advanced fitness program. The last part of the book focuses on nutrition and my plan for those who want to go all the way. Yes, we're going to get results, so don't sweat that part of it . . . but you *will* be doing plenty of sweating—I promise!

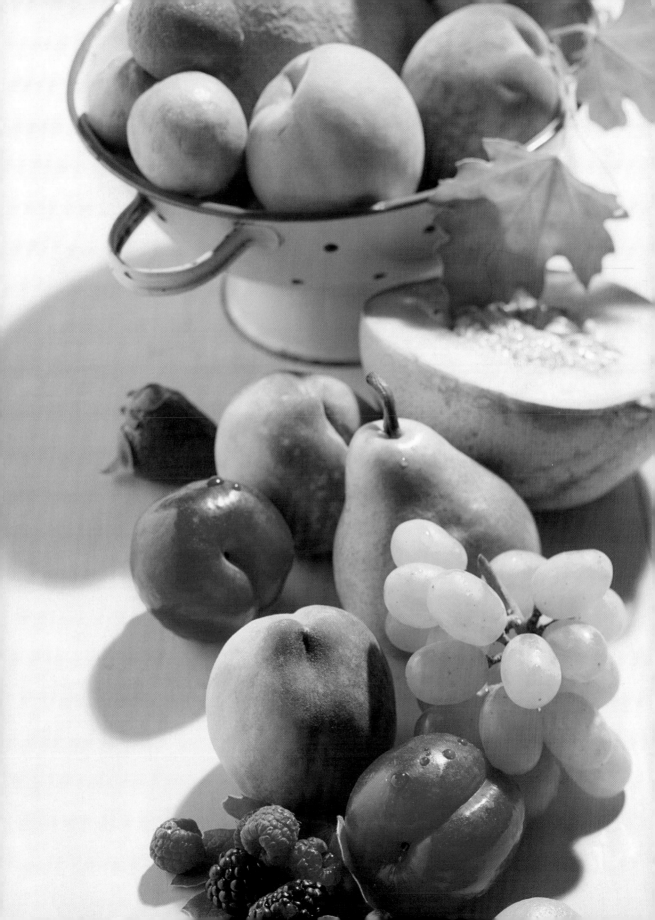

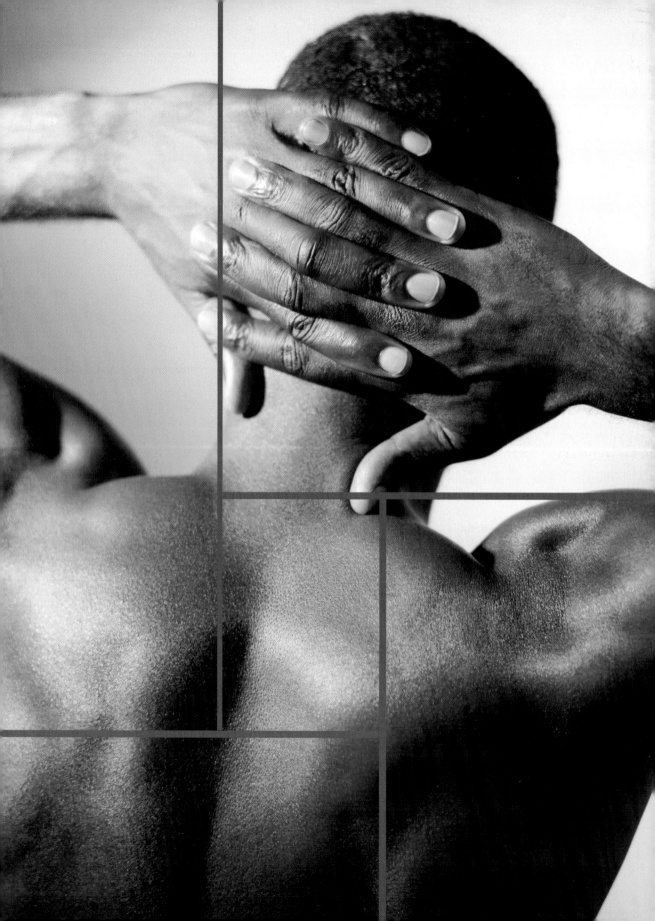

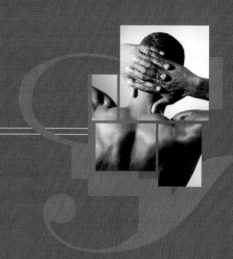

PART I
Getting Ready for The TRUTH

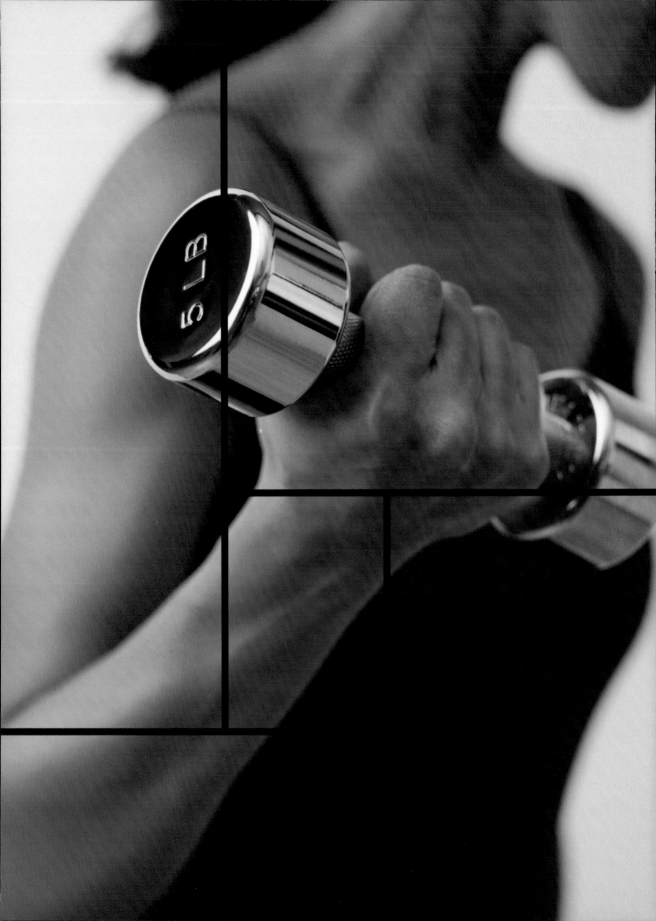

WHAT *IS* THE TRUTH?

Welcome to The TRUTH program. I'm here to give you some honest answers when it comes to training techniques, optimal nutrition, the power of cardio, and the effectiveness of weight training. Of course, when we get done, the ultimate answer will stare back at you in the mirror. You'll experience the joy of having the body of your dreams.

Before we begin, let me tell you what The TRUTH means to me, and why it's the most empowering program you can embark on. I promise that the real power of The TRUTH—indeed, its very effectiveness—lies in its sheer simplicity.

T: The **T**ime is Now!

You have to decide that there's no time like the present to start on an effective fitness program and make a healthy commitment to your body, your self-esteem, and your longevity.

R: **R**eality Check

I'll identify the most common fitness myths and misconceptions that might have stopped you from seeing the results you want from a health-and-fitness program. It's not that you've necessarily been doing something wrong, but what you've been doing may have been wrong for your body.

U: **U**nleash Your Mental Power

A proper program goes much deeper than just getting your body in shape—it begins with your mind and making a commitment to a new lifestyle. I'll help you flex your brainpower to set realistic goals and find the power within your body. I'll set you up for success, and then keep you motivated, positive, and on track.

T: **T**rain, Train, Train

Now that we've got your head on straight, I'll teach you the proper weight-training and cardiovascular exercises for your current state of fitness. Whether you've never stepped foot in a gym or have trained for years, you'll find a program that's perfect for you, one that will advance you to the next level.

H: **H**ealthy Eating

The final component to The TRUTH is a meal plan in which you can eat healthy foods that work hand-in-hand with your training program to help you look and feel fantastic. I'll tell you how to make the best choices at the supermarket, at a restaurant, and at your own dining-room table. Almost everyone I meet is totally confused about proper eating, but who can blame them? It seems as if every single day there's a new diet philosophy out there that promises to give you all the answers. My program is easy to understand and follow. (P.S.: You'll love my special cheat meals that will help keep you sane, boost your metabolism, and make it easier to stay on track.)

The bottom line is that The TRUTH *is* the truth when it comes to unlocking your physical and mental potential and achieving a state of happiness and fulfillment. I know it's possible because the dream came true for me. The program has also worked for my clients—men and women ranging from 18 to 73 years old. I'm talking celebrities, pro athletes, stay-at-home moms, business professionals, and students. So, if you're asking if The TRUTH has ever worked for "someone like me," the answer is yes.

I know you're probably saying, "Frank, you've never met me, and I've already been on approximately 374 diets that have failed. Why is your plan going to be any different?"

First of all, The TRUTH respects genetic differences and varying levels of fitness experience. It isn't a one-size-fits-all program that fails to recognize that everyone is different and needs his or her own unique fitness plan. I've designed weight-training, cardiovascular, and nutritional programs that will allow anyone to immediately get started on the road to a new body—and a new life.

Whether you're in excellent shape already and want to look and feel even better, or you've never touched a weight in your life and need to lose a few dozen pounds, you'll absolutely find a starting point to achieving your goals in this book. I've made it easy because I know where most people fail on their fitness plan: They try to follow one blueprint for nutrition, strength training, and cardio.

With The TRUTH, you get to identify three separate levels, and turn them into one plan that works for you on all fronts. Stick with me for a minute here. For example, maybe you're a Level 2 nutrition person because you're great at cutting out fat, but you're a Level 1 when it comes to cardio because the treadmill in your bedroom is under four inches of dust, yet you're pretty strong and can start weight lifting at Level 2. That's why I'd start you at a few different levels, which will equal one successful plan. Maybe another person will follow Level 3 weight training, Level 2 cardio, and Level 1 eating for the first 30 days. Bear with me, and this will be a cinch.

Take a look at the five levels of strength training, and you'll understand what I mean. Later, I'll fill you in on the different levels when it comes to cardio and nutrition. But first, let's help you get stronger.

Level 1: This is the beginner's level, which has been designed for people who have never picked up a weight in their life. You'll learn how to perform some basic movements, get the blood flowing, and wake up those muscles that haven't been used in a while (if ever). This is the ultimate beginner's circuit-training program that will yield great results while motivating you to get to the next level.

Level 2: This level has been designed for people who lift occasionally or have tried other beginner programs with mixed (or absolutely no) results. This program is a bit more advanced than the Level 1 circuit-training program and will allow you to work on each body part.

Level 3: This is for intermediate weight trainers who have been on another program for too long and need a new challenge to achieve even greater results. Some of you may graduate to this level after Levels 1 and 2, while others might start at this level because of past experience. I'll help you combine key primary exercises for each important area of your body, plus we'll add new, exciting secondary exercises that will put that extra polish on your new physique.

Level 4: This is a more advanced routine for those who have graduated from the first three levels. It's also for those people who've been seriously training for years and really want to push it. Give me the same dedication and commitment that you've always brought to the gym, and I'll help you truly create the body of your dreams. I'll cover all the advanced exercises that will refine your body, and bring it to a level of true greatness.

Level 5: Just when you think I've pushed you to the limit, there's one more step. This is where we'll go wild, and I'll introduce the secrets I've never revealed before to keep your body at a maximum level. We'll also work on keeping workouts fresh, fun, and effective. I'll eliminate the sheer boredom and monotony of doing the same old workout again and again. This motivation killer will be a thing of the past, so you can maintain what we'll achieve together.

Of course, there are some common denominators for all the levels, and these include the stretching, cardio, and nutrition tips that I'll tell you about in upcoming chapters. All you have to do is select the weight-training, cardio, and nutrition levels that seem right for you, and go for it! You can't make a mistake, because if you try Level 3 and it's just too much for you, well, just slip into Level 2 and work up to your "promotion" when the time seems right.

There's no such thing as failure when you're into The TRUTH. You'll work at your own pace and graduate to the next level when your body says so.

I don't believe in making people feel guilty because they aren't ready to make as big of a commitment as somebody else is. The fact that you're ready to make *any* commitment today is a step in the right direction. Congratulations!

Now let's get your mind moving when it comes to the motivational part of the journey. It's truly the first step.

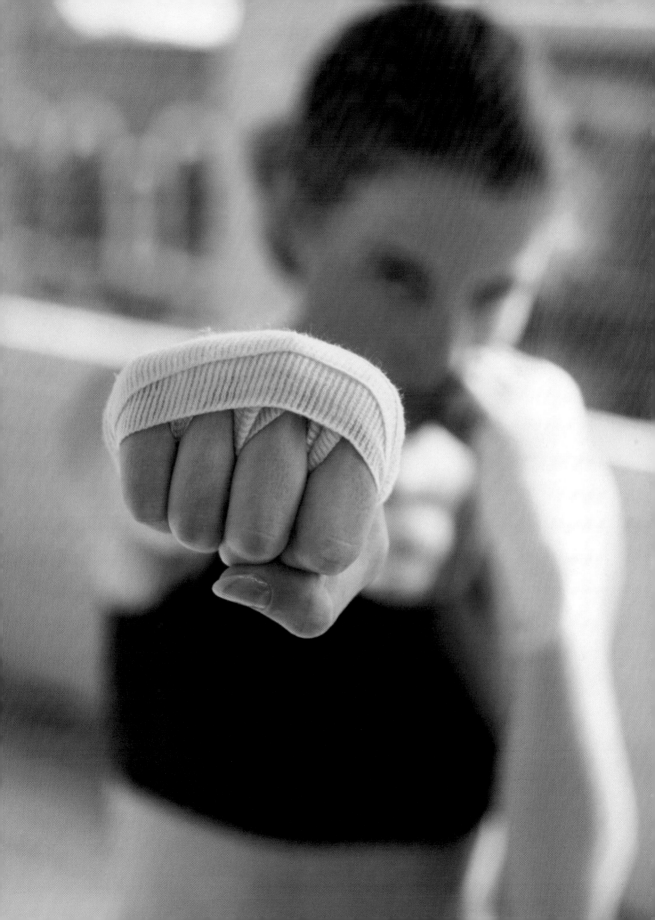

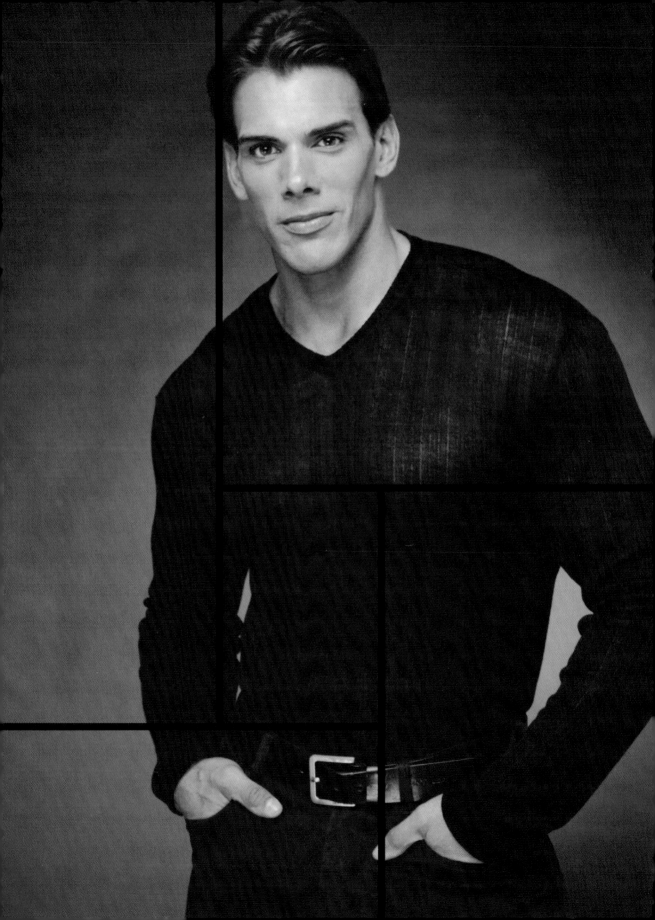

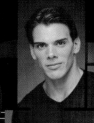

C H A P T E R   2

THE MENTAL WORKOUT

One of the challenges I knew I'd be facing when I started to write this book was how to get my new client (that means you) to make a serious commitment to fitness and health. Let's face facts: The two hardest aspects of working on yourself are getting started and sticking with it.

Hey, if this stuff was easy, we'd all walk around looking like we just got home from a tough day posing for *GQ* or *In Style*. Or in this same dreamworld, lifting a two-liter bottle of Coke to a glass would be considered working on our biceps.

I hate to be a downer, but what keeps me motivated is fear. I've spoken with many medical professionals who've explained to me that the negative effects of being overweight and out of shape are enormous, frightening, and quite serious. In other words, it goes way beyond feeling bad or not fitting into our favorite jeans.

If you're still not convinced, and would rather sit on the couch curled up with a bag of chips and the remote control, ask yourself the following questions:

"Am I willing to risk becoming another statistic?" I know you're probably saying, "Thanks, Frank—I just want to hide under the covers and not even think about that one." But the sad truth is that if you're overweight, you have a greater risk of experiencing serious, life-threatening ailments including heart disease, diabetes, lung conditions, cancer, skeletal problems, and so on. Denial isn't going to make the statistics go away, no matter how much I wish it would.

"If I continue to live in this unhealthy way, what will happen to me in five years? Will my life be better or worse? Will I even be alive?" Yeah, I know that's really a scary thought, but there are some people who truly need to mull this over. I can't give you the answer. All I know is that if you keep abusing your body, you'll eventually pay the price. It's inevitable.

The better you care for yourself, the longer you'll live; consequently, your quality of life will be that much sweeter. That's one truth we can all agree on.

Now, I'd like to give you a few quick statistics to ponder:

- Approximately 127 million American adults are overweight. That translates to almost two of every three adults in the U.S. being overweight.

- An estimated 60 million American adults are obese, nearly one of every three. And nine million are considered severely obese.

- Obesity causes at least 300,000 deaths per year in the U.S.

- Health-care costs for obese American adults can run up to $100 billion per year.

Now do I have your attention? Good. Let's continue with our question-and-answer session:

"Okay, now I'm a little worried. Can't we just fix me, and fast?" I wish I could give you a quick plan that melts off the pounds in a month and sends you on your way, but if I *did* make that promise, then this book would be called *The LIE.*

Have you ever wondered why, if all those miracle products and fad diets that we've heard about over the years worked, all the statistics about weight and obesity have just gotten worse? Obviously, whatever is being sold to us isn't getting the job done.

"Fine, I'll stay away from quick fixes. But why do I keep gaining weight? I don't really pig out that much, and I try to exercise." First, you should give yourself a break—our lifestyles in the 21st century are very conducive to packing on the pounds. Today we live in an era of convenience, which has its pluses and minuses. I mean, I'm glad that I don't have to go out into the wilderness and hunt a turkey in order to get in a little protein at dinner. (After all, I'd probably just catch the turkey and adopt him as a pet while starving to death.) Then again, it's not so great that I can get in my car to drive to the supermarket, where I can stuff myself with millions of convenience foods. Even worse is the fact that I can pull up to any fast-food joint in America and instantly receive 1,000-plus empty calories to shove down my throat.

But our food choices only make up part of the equation. I can just imagine how many calories women once burned beating clothes on a rock to get them clean. Plus, think of all that great stretching! These days we just drive to the dry cleaners and lift the pile of clothes from the trunk of our cars, walk two steps, and get out the checkbook. You get the idea. We need to go back to the basics: clean, good food and moving, moving, moving.

"Now I'm convinced that I have to do 'something,' but I honestly don't have the time to follow some involved program." Hey, I feel your pain. Getting in shape takes time, effort, and perseverance, so you've really got to commit to making the time to get it done. Of course most people want immediate results and instant gratification—when they don't see the expected results in a short time, they quit and go seek the two-minute-a-day workout plan. Then the same people figure, "Well, I don't really have two minutes either."

I can promise you that if you devote a reasonable amount of time to practicing The TRUTH, you're going to see the kind of results that will make you want to stick with it. And without even realizing it at first, you'll begin to change your entire way of life. I think you'll enjoy the process, so the time spent will be worthwhile.

There isn't a person on this earth who is honestly too busy to exercise. Go to your local gym and you'll see a diverse group of people who finds the time to work out: single moms, business professionals, and grandparents. Even the President of the United States has time to get moving.

I firmly believe that everyone can make the time if it's important enough to them. After all, what's more important than your health? Not much. So make it your top priority.

"This all sounds great, but my stomach looks like a doughy mountain, and I can barely walk to the corner without huffing and puffing. In other words, I'm seriously out of shape. Now what?" First of all, you're not alone. As I mentioned before, two out of every three American adults walking around are overweight and out of shape. That's why I've geared my beginner's program (Level 1) to people who have never worked out in their lives. By just getting in the game, you'll find that you'll love the results.

"I hate myself for being overweight. Is that normal?" The emotional baggage of being overweight can be truly crushing. Your fat can consciously affect your daily thought processes, self-esteem, and behavior, as well as your relationships with others. If you don't feel good about yourself and don't have confidence in your appearance and/or health, *everything* in your life will be impacted. If you're overweight and content, I'm still worried about your health, but I'm happy for you. However, most overweight people tell me that they have a cloud of unhappiness that follows them around all day, from which there is no escape.

The TRUTH program has a funny way of making feel people better because they're finally taking some control of the situation. Just one day of eating correctly and working out will mean that you accomplished something major. Think about the satisfaction and pride you'll feel as you wake up tomorrow, ready to seize the day and all that the world has to offer.

I only hope that you're as excited as I am to unleash the new you to the world!

Taking Stock: The TRUTH Happiness Percentage ("THP")

Now that you realize the potential of what we're about to accomplish together, along with what's really at stake, it's time for you to answer some difficult questions. And please be honest with yourself. Your personal truths may hurt a little bit, but The TRUTH is going to help you change all those feelings.

Before we put you on that path, you have to consciously acknowledge and realize where you are today. In order to do that, I need you to stand up and get a pencil or pen. (See how I'm starting out by going easy on you?)

On a scale of 1 to 10, 1 being "totally disagree" and 10 being "totally agree," I want you to assign a number to each of the following statements. I'd also like you to place today's date at the top.

THP for:

[insert date]

NUMBER (1–10):   **QUESTIONS**

_____ 1. When I look at myself in the mirror without clothes on, I feel positive, confident, and happy.

_____ 2. When I look at myself in the mirror with my favorite outfit on, I feel positive, confident, and happy.

_____ 3. When I think about going to the beach in a revealing bathing suit, I look forward to getting there.

_____ 4. When I think about going shopping for clothes, I'm eager to try on different outfits and see how I'll look in them.

_____ 5. When I think about having sex with the lights on, it's exciting, and I know that I'll turn my partner on. I feel no shame in how I look, and I'm not self-conscious at all.

_____ 6. I'm confident that I'm living a lifestyle that will keep me as healthy as possible and add years to my life.

_____ 7. My current appearance and fitness lifestyle enhances my interpersonal relationships with family, friends, significant others, and co-workers.

_____ 8. My current appearance enhances these aspects of my life: mental and emotional stability, work performance, and an active social life.

_____ 9. When I make an appointment to see the doctor, I don't fear that the way I've been living my life will reveal any negative health issues.

_____ 10. I'm truly happy.

_____ TOTAL

To Figure Out Your Score or THP: Add up your numbers. This is your TRUTH Happiness Percentage or "THP." If you scored a 53, for example, your THP is currently 53 percent. I recommend that you go back and re-take the test at three-month intervals after you begin following The TRUTH to see how your THP changes every few months.

If you're true to the program, you'll be amazed at how your personal THP climbs toward higher and higher levels of fulfillment and contentment. It's a good and easy way to monitor your progress.

One More Thing about Motivating Yourself

Repeat after me: "*Now*—not next week or next month." You don't have to wait until next Monday morning to start this program, or next month or next year. The only thing that will be different if you wait is that you'll be in worse condition than you are today. You'll have to work harder and longer to reach your goals because waiting will mean that you just have further to go.

The alternative to taking immediate action and getting on a positive fitness path is to do nothing and simply accept your current condition. So do you want to become another statistic, or will you choose to be a success story?

We're in this together—and since my goal is to get everyone who reads this book in better shape, I need your help. I really want you to succeed.

I've saved this info for now just in case you need a final push: Consider that if you lose just 10 percent of your body weight and keep it off, you can decrease your chances of being affected by many less-than-desirable medical conditions, while improving your overall appearance and health profile at the same time. Now that's a true win-win situation.

Still Have a Few Excuses?

If I had a nickel for every excuse I've heard in the past ten years, I'd be living in a castle on my own Mediterranean island. I think that the number-one reason people don't accomplish their goals is that they make excuses. It's not because they *can't* do it, it's because they *won't*. You're going to have to think up a few new ones, because I've heard some of the best excuses in the book:

- *I don't have the time to work out—I'm too busy.*

- *I have kids. Running after them is my workout.*

- *The gym is too far away from home, so I don't have time to go there and back.*

- *I work all day—how can I eat healthy foods?*

- *It's too expensive to eat nutritious meals.*

- *I can't eat four or five times a day!*

- *I don't like the gym. The people annoy me.*

- *I don't want to drink protein shakes—I hear they give you liver damage.*

- *I'll get too muscular if I lose weight.*

- *I'm not a narcissist, so why should I work out?*

Do you know what all of these excuses have in common? They're lies that will stop you from becoming the person you always wanted to be—the person you *can* be.

JUST IN CASE YOU HAVE any self-limiting fitness myths rolling around in your head that may be holding you back from putting your heart into your commitment to The TRUTH, don't worry. Once you read the next chapter, that sort of thinking will become a thing of the past.

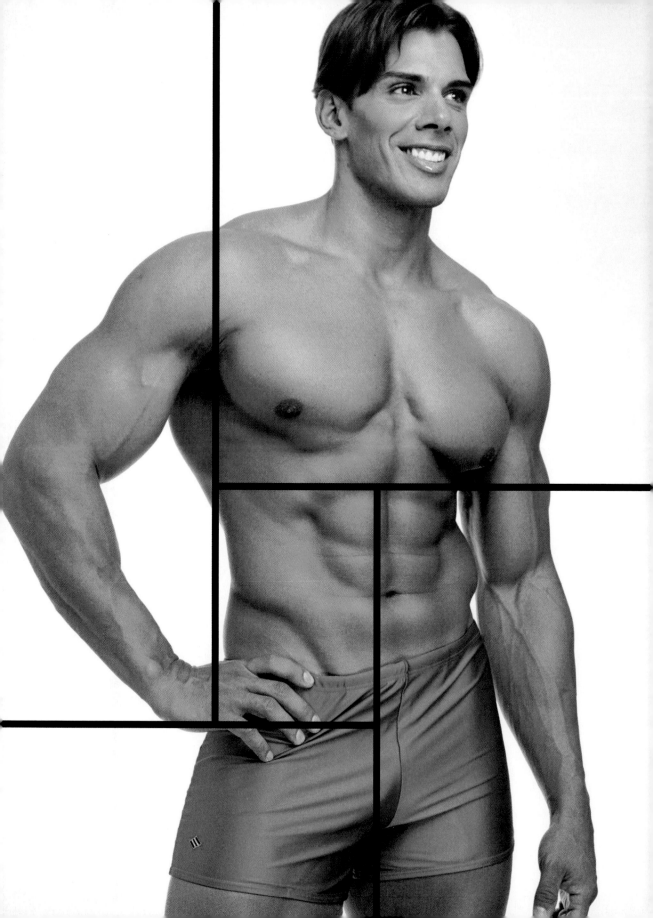

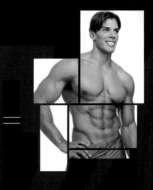

C H A P T E R　3

MY FAVORITE FITNESS MYTHS

So many fitness myths, so little time. . . .

Here's an example of what I mean. A few years ago, a woman at the gym motioned me over to her. "Frank, I have to ask you something about those barbells in the corner," she whispered conspiratorially.

I leaned in, thinking this was going to be a whopper.

"If I lift weights, will my arms grow longer? I really can't afford to buy specialty blouses."

Through my laughter, I assured her, "That's just a fitness myth. Your arms will grow stronger, but certainly not longer!"

It really wasn't this woman's fault. After all, the misinformation about fitness runs very deep. Some of these myths are funny, while others revolve around some legitimate concerns. But sadly, they all share one thing in common: They stop a lot of people from committing to a healthy lifestyle program.

Following are the most common fitness myths I've heard over the years, along with the facts that correspond to them.

Myth: "I don't know the right way to work out, and I can't afford a personal trainer, so I guess I can't really do any exercise program."

Reality Check: That might have been an excuse before today, but since you're holding *The TRUTH* in your hands, you're also holding full access to a professional personal trainer! The good news is that you paid less for this book than many people pay to spend a half an hour with a trainer like myself. You'll also be able to look at photos of me performing each of the exercises, so you can learn the proper form for each move. And while most trainers won't give you an eating plan, later on in the book I'll get to several eating (not *starving*) programs, which will help you attain your goals.

Myth: "Gyms and health clubs are for people who are already in shape. I don't want people to stare at me or think I don't belong."

Reality Check: First, you must realize that everyone starts somewhere. People aren't born in the gym with six-pack abs or huge biceps protruding from their tank tops.

Next, I'll let you in on a little secret. Most people who are in shape and make the gym a regular part of their healthy lifestyle respect one thing in fellow members: serious effort. I know that when I see overweight members at my gym working hard, I think, *I'm really proud of those people for making the effort because it's not easy. I'm glad that they're trying to better themselves.*

Myth: "It's too expensive to get in shape. We're talking gym memberships and buying the right food, not to mention those cool workout outfits. I just can't afford it."

Reality Check: As we discussed in the previous chapter, it's more expensive to be *out* of shape. Think of your doctor bills. And gym memberships are being offered for as little as $15 a month, which is less than the cost of one prescription for high blood pressure—much less. It's also cheaper than going to McDonald's a few times a month.

Myth: "To lose weight and get in great shape, I'll have to practically starve myself to death. But maybe that would be a good thing—after all, the less I eat, the more quickly I'll get in shape."

Reality Check: I promise that you won't be starving on my program. Believe it or not, most diets fail because they're too low in calories. What happens is that your body initially drops some weight because of the limited calories. However, your metabolism consequently slows down, so this low-calorie diet is now exactly what your body needs to maintain your current weight—meaning that you're not losing poundage anymore. After a few weeks of starving and failing to lose weight (or possibly even gaining some), you start to eat more. Who wouldn't? And now you're part of a club that has millions of members: the yo-yo diet club.

The TRUTH nutritional program will help you build—not destroy—your metabolism. You'll earn how to eat correctly without starving your body of what it needs to keep yielding great results.

Myth: "If I exercise, then I'll be able to eat whatever I want and won't gain weight, right?"

Reality Check: Don't hate me, but no. Unfortunately, exercising doesn't give you a license to cheat. If losing weight is your goal, then you have to keep a very simple equation in mind: *The calories you burn must exceed the calories you take in.* For example, let's say that you eat everything on your diet plan, but thanks to old habits, you add a few tasty treats in, such as a little frozen yogurt, a handful of potato chips, and a slice of pizza. Well, you've just added more than *1,000* calories to your plan. If you work out to burn 700 calories, those extra 300 calories still have to go somewhere—they'll add up and settle on your hips, abs, and butt.

Myth: "If I eat more than I eat now, then I'm just going to get fatter."

Reality Check: Of course that *can* be true, but not if you eat what I've outlined for you in the nutrition portion of this book. Again, it all comes down to calories burned versus calories eaten. We're going to eat good food and then burn off the calories. You'll constantly be fueling your body and firing up your metabolism. And while you'll almost definitely be eating more food, it doesn't mean that your calorie intake will be greater than it is now. Think *quality over quantity.*

Myth: "As a woman, I shouldn't exercise with weights—otherwise I'll start looking like one of those female bodybuilders."

Reality Check: Wrong. This is actually my favorite myth. As a personal trainer, I have many female clients, and the one recurring theme with most of them is, "I want a program that builds muscle, but I don't want to be as big as you." Bottom line: It's impossible for a woman who starts training with weights and does so on a regular basis to get a physique like mine.

Building muscle is a very gradual process. The only way that a woman can build huge muscles is by using hormones and steroids. On the other hand, I feel that the right amount of muscle on a woman is very feminine, attractive, and sexy. I love the toned look of Janet Jackson, Demi Moore, and Angelina Jolie. Don't worry about getting too big—just worry about getting in shape.

Myth: "I'm a man who worries that if I work out with weights, I'll get musclebound, thus limiting my flexibility."

Reality Check: Don't worry. You won't wake up one morning looking like a candidate for Mr. Olympia. And the idea that muscles will limit flexibility is an old wives' tale that has been completely discredited by fitness experts. Years ago, athletes such as boxers, golfers, and basketball and baseball players were forbidden to touch weights for fear they'd become "musclebound" and lose the flexibility required to be successful in their chosen sport. Keep in mind that they also used to tell athletes not to have sex before a game. Boy, how things have changed. Now it would be impossible to find a top athlete who doesn't incorporate weight training into his or her conditioning program (and don't even get me started on the sex!).

Myth: "If I start working out and then stop, my muscles will turn into a mass of fat."

Reality Check: When was the last time you saw an overweight person walking down the street and said, "He better be careful—all that fat is going to turn into muscle and then he'll be really musclebound"? It's medically impossible for muscle to turn to fat, because muscle and fat are completely different types of tissue and can't miraculously turn into the other. What sometimes happens is that a person will stop working out but will continue to eat as much food as they did when they were active. So they gain weight, while the muscles developed during training get smaller. That's why it might look as if their muscles have "turned to fat"—but they haven't. In other words, when you stop working out, your body simply takes on a softer and smaller look.

Myth: "Weight training won't help me get leaner, it will only make my muscles bigger."

Reality Check: Working out with weights will help you get leaner all over for a few reasons. First, when you have more muscle tissue, your metabolism speeds up, causing you to burn more calories than you eat, which will give you a leaner body. Second, when you weight-train, your body tends to burn a specific type of food: carbohydrates, which are usually the food source people binge on. Coincidentally, carbs are also what the body burns first when you weight-train. So, by adding weight training into your overall fitness approach with The TRUTH, you'll burn more of the very food source that you need to burn.

Myth: "If I start one of those programs in the magazines or on TV, I'll look like the people in the ads in record time."

Reality Check: Most of those ads are just plain ridiculous. The Federal Trade Commission has even hit some of these companies with a huge fine when it was discovered that they were using computer-generated before-and-after photos. So maybe the spokesmodel said she lost an incredible 30 pounds in 30 days—but in reality, she lost mostly water weight and not fat . . . if she really lost anything at all. You see, it's almost impossible to lose more than two pounds of fat per week. By setting yourself up with unrealistic, false, and unhealthy expectations, you'll get derailed from your success, and I don't want that to happen to you again.

Myth: "If I use an ab machine, I'll be lean and have a great midsection in no time."

Reality Check: The next time your favorite ab machine is advertised on TV, tape the commercial. Then rewind the tape and read the fine print at the end. You'll see nice little letters on the bottom of the screen that say something such as "results not typical" and "when used in conjunction with a diet-and-exercise program." Do you know what that means? You can do 5,000 repetitions a day on your spanking new machine, but you're not going to have the body of the guy or girl in the commercial. Sorry.

Myth: "If I take one of those fat-loss pills I hear about all the time, I'll lose weight without having to exercise or watch what I eat. Plus, I see them in the health-food store, so they must be safe."

Reality Check: You can probably answer this one yourself by now—*there's no such thing as a magic pill.* Unfortunately, many people are finding out the hard way that these popular fat-burning supplements contain ephedrine, ephedra, and ma huang, all of which can be very dangerous. These ingredients are central nervous system (CNS) stimulants and have been linked to serious health problems involving the heart. There have been numerous deaths linked to CNS stimulants, and there's a strong movement toward banning these substances altogether. The TRUTH is about making you healthier, risk free. It's that simple.

Myth: "If I just stay on the treadmill or another piece of cardio equipment long enough, I'll get in great shape."

Reality Check: Again, the principle that calories burned should exceed calories consumed applies if you're trying to lose weight. If you take in 1,000 calories and do an hour of cardio a day, you won't be in great shape, I'm afraid. You must perform the cardio at the correct intensity to get the desired result. If you go too slowly, you're not going to get much out of the activity; move too fast and you'll end up burning muscle instead of unwanted fat. Using The TRUTH, you'll learn how to determine your optimal cardiovascular performance level. I'll give you a few proven program levels to choose from in a later chapter.

Also, how do you expect to sculpt and build muscle by running on the treadmill? The answer is you can't. You have to do a *complete* program that also contains weight-resistance exercises.

Myth: "I'm not strong enough to lift heavy barbells."

Reality Check: You don't have to lift tremendous amounts of weight to get results. Muscle tissue is made up of two types of fibers called "slow twitch" and "fast twitch." One is most responsive when stimulated with higher repetitions using lighter weights, while the other is most responsive to lower repetitions with heavier weight. Therefore, when you use lighter weights for higher reps, you'll be stimulating fast-twitch fibers and increasing muscle tissue. And you'll be doing it without the use of any heavy weight. Consistency is key. Higher-repetition programs with lighter weights create a higher level of muscle tone and a more refined, polished-looking physique. Now, that's good news!

Myth: "I can't lift weights and do cardio in the same day. That's too much for my poor body to handle!"

Reality Check: Eating fast food, drinking beer, and sitting on the sofa watching TV all day is too much for the body to handle! Weight training and cardio are both necessary in order to create the physique you want—when done together, they work synergistically to build and sculpt muscle (with a proper diet). There's no reason why you can't do them on the same day because you're taking advantage of the different types of positive, result-producing activities.

Myth: "This is sort of an embarrassing one, but I heard that weight training will make a guy's genitals smaller. True or false? (God, I hope it's false.)"

Reality Check: Okay, I gotta stop laughing here . . . wait, I can't stop! Seriously, I think this myth was started by a guy who lost his girlfriend to a bodybuilder. All I can say is that if the family jewels were in jeopardy, weight rooms at gyms across the nation would be empty. They seem pretty full to me, so that's just one way of saying that this is hogwash. But again, thanks for the laugh.

Myth: "Once I reach my goals, I can stop working out and go back to my old lifestyle."

Reality Check: You *could* go back, I guess, but why? Why would you want to erase all of the hard work you've invested in yourself? The TRUTH program is a lifestyle that will keep you strong and lean over the long haul, *if* you set your mind on these goals. The next chapter will help you tone up that gray matter.

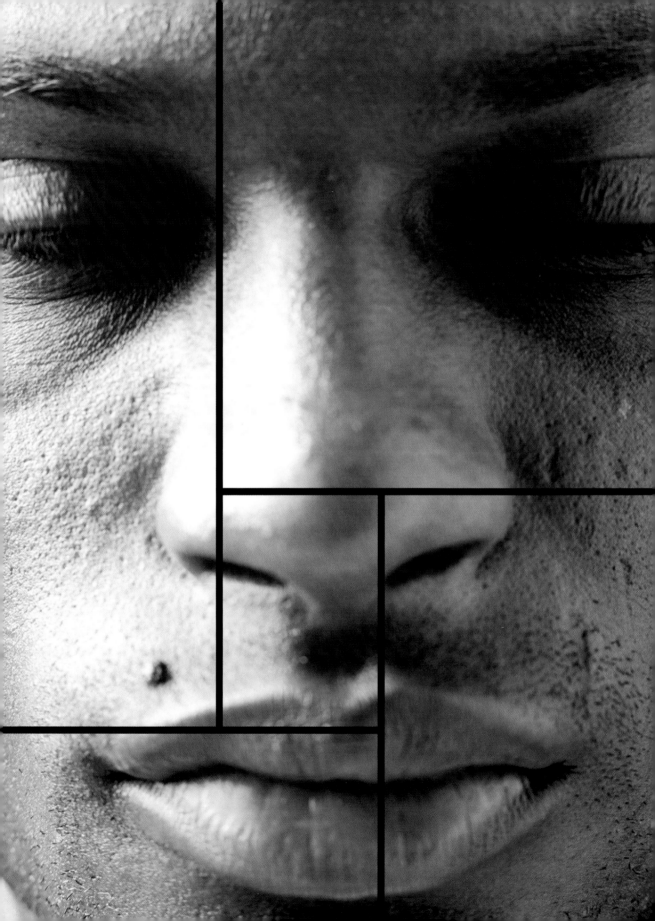

CHAPTER 4

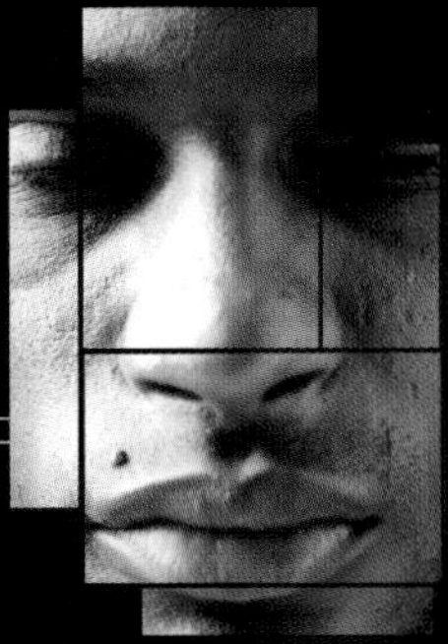

UNLEASH YOUR MENTAL POWER

Now's the time for you to make good on all those promises you keep making to yourself. You know the ones I'm talking about: *This year I'm going to lose 20 pounds. I'm going to go to the beach without being embarrassed by my body. I will get in the best shape of my life.*

Well, guess what? You can finally do all of the above!

In this chapter, I'll give you the appropriate mental tools to help you define your goals, stay motivated, and put The TRUTH into action. Since the mind dictates what the body's going to do, they both have to be in sync if this program is going to work for you.

It's time to begin to unleash your power by strengthening your mental capacity. Let's get started!

Step 1: Set a Fitness Goal

If you listen to any self-help guru or motivational speaker, they'll tell you the same thing: *To be successful, you first have to set goals.* Most of us already do this thousands of times a day. For example, we make sure that the bills are paid and there's food in the house. I mean, we don't believe that food will just magically appear on our table when we get home—our goal is to go out and buy it.

On the other hand, I rarely hear people set goals when it comes to fitness. They just want "to get skinny" or "become toned." Unfortunately, a goal to lose weight or get in shape won't cut it because they aren't goals; they're wishes or dreams.

I need you to set a *specific* goal. In other words, how many pounds do you want to lose by what specific date? The only way you're going to know if you've reached your goal is if you're definite about it. A vague goal without a time frame attached to it won't help you get up tomorrow morning and take action. So I want you to say, "I will lose [fill in the blank] pounds of body fat in the next [fill in the blank] weeks." You can also frame your goal this way: "I will lose 15 percent of my body fat by July 15." If weight loss isn't what you're trying to do, then you need to set goals that incorporate your commitment to The TRUTH. You might say, "I will follow Level 3 weight training, Level 2 cardio, and Level 1 eating for the next 30 days. After 30 days, I'm going to move to the next level."

Once you've gotten specific, it will be easier to head toward your goal because you'll know exactly what you want to accomplish, *and* you'll have a firm deadline that will push you to get the most out of your exercise and nutrition programs.

Before we get started, I'd like to clarify that I want you to set challenging yet reasonable goals. It's not going to cut it if you announce, "I'm going to lose 70 pounds in 30 days," "I'm going to bench-press 1,000 pounds by next week," or "I know I'm 50 pounds overweight, but I'm going to be featured on the cover of *Vogue* in three months." Here you're just setting yourself up to fail, which is only going to make you feel worse and rock your self-esteem and confidence. The idea is to feel better about yourself.

Here's an example to illustrate what I'm talking about here. My client Patty was getting married, so she said, "Frank, I don't care what you do with me. You have to help me melt off 20 pounds of lard in three months. I also want some muscle tone because I bought an off-the-shoulder dress." Is this reasonable and attainable? Well, I told Patty that she could achieve her goals by following The TRUTH training and nutritional programs. She could shed the body fat and tone up if she paid careful attention to weight training, cardio, and a nutritional plan. *Hold it–20 pounds in three months?* I can hear you thinking. *Is this possible?* Absolutely. Remember, I told you before that you can expect to lose two pounds a week, or eight pounds a month. So, let's do the math: If Patty gives herself three months, that's plenty of time to lose 20 pounds of fat and tone up.

Patty's goal is actually pretty good because it's reasonable and challenging. In other words, there's nothing that can stop Patty from getting into that beautiful dress of her dreams—except herself.

Step 2: Stop Comparing Yourself to Everyone (or Anyone) Else

You may find it motivating to think of Jennifer Aniston and say, "I want her body someday," but let's get real. You need to commit to having *your* best body. That means that you need to follow your own individual program and forget about what your best friend or the lady down the street is doing. Just because Angie from carpool is following that "eat-grapefruit-all-day diet" and she lost ten pounds last week (of water weight, and it's really not ten pounds, but about three), that doesn't mean you should follow suit. You have to personalize your nutrition-and-workout plan to your level of fitness and genetic makeup. The only person you should be competing against is yourself.

Step 3: Write Down Your Goals

Your mind is capable of many great things, but it's not a notebook. Goals that are kept in your head can float in and out of your consciousness. And when those objectives seem too tough, you can just put them out of your mind. That's why I want you to commit your goals to writing, which causes you to make a more substantial commitment than simply telling yourself that you'll "do something." Once you write them down, your goals become real, verifiable, and not so easily forgotten. It's harder to quit when you have a written record.

I know a guy named Fred who was substantially overweight when I met him. Months later, and after a lot of hard work, he'd lost 50 pounds.

"Fred, what was so different this time?" I asked this man, who had been on every diet under the sun.

"Well, I pulled out one sheet of notebook paper and wrote down my goals," he told me. "On the top, I put a photo of the fat me. Then I taped the whole thing to my refrigerator door. Every time I wanted to binge, I'd see that old picture and read my goals. I found that I could walk away from having a snack I didn't need." Fred went on to explain that this small, simple task had given him the kind of commitment that he never found with any other approach to diet and exercise.

Step 4: Commit to Both Short-Term and Long-Term Goals

Now that you understand how to set empowering, action-producing objectives, I recommend that you set both short- and long-term goals. When it comes to long-term goals, pretend that you're a marathon runner at the beginning of the most exciting race of your life. As you stand at the starting line, you can see that your long-term goal might be to lose 30 pounds of fat, replace it with muscle, and sculpt some of those fantastic six-pack abs. That's a great goal, and one that will take some time to achieve—like running a marathon. But if you begin with a few simple steps in the right direction, those will make up your short-term goals. Long-term goals are so far off in the future that it's easy for us to get started "next week," "next month," or "next millennium." What's the rush? Short-term goals, on the other hand, require immediate attention, and that's the real way to get off your tush and start The TRUTH.

Your short-term goals should never be more than three months in duration because you should feel as if there's a sense of urgency in achieving them. If you give yourself five months to lose 15 pounds, for example, you can always start tomorrow—in other words, you have plenty of time to achieve that goal. There's no need to commit to your program right away. However, if you give yourself a shorter but reasonable time frame, then your commitment will be strong and you'll be able to achieve your objective immediately.

Personally, I like to set short-term goals every 30 days because this time frame allows me to see both physical and mental changes in myself. I think it's important to emotionally know that you're moving in a positive direction. If you can see that you're making progress, then you'll remain encouraged and stay on the path. Plus, if you aren't getting the results you hoped for, you can just make the necessary changes in your diet and workout program to get you right back on the correct path.

My client Louie had never been in a gym during his 45 years on this planet, but as he told me, "I dream of having the body of Adonis. I want every girl to notice me when I walk by." I had to smile because I admire a man who shoots for the moon! Now the reality of this situation was that Louie weighed 205 pounds and had a 20-percent body-fat level. I knew (and so did he) that we had to get rid of a significant amount of body fat and gain quite a bit of lean muscle for him to turn into that kind of girl magnet.

Within a year of healthy eating, weight training, and regular cardio workouts, Louie only had 10-percent body fat. He now also sports a toned physique and shows off a solid set of abs. But in order to get to this place, Louie had to set several short-term goals beyond wishing to be Adonis. His first goal was to lose 15 pounds in three months and complete the first two levels of The TRUTH. Mission accomplished. His next three-month goal was to lose 12 more pounds and complete Level 3 of the program. Again, he sailed right past his second short-term goal. And as he reached each milestone, Louie would say, "Frank, I've never felt better in my life."

At the end of our first six months together, Louie had shed 27 pounds and was almost done with Level 3. That meant he was halfway to his long-term goal, which would take one year to complete. This might never have happened if Louie hadn't set that first short-term goal to lose 15 pounds in three months. That step made him start *now,* instead of next week or next month.

Achieving your long-term goals is only a matter of successfully completing a series of short-term goals along the way. This not only applies to your body, but to the rest of your goals in life as well. (Hey, I won't bill you for the extra therapy!)

Step 5: Stay Positively Motivated

You're probably going to have a bad day, or maybe even a few bad days in a row, where you fall off your program. Your motivation will start to wane a little bit, and suddenly you'll be thinking about giving up or giving in to more behavior that will keep you further away from your goals. Please come back to this chapter when that happens and know that I've had bad days, too. I've even been known to eat a little chocolate-chip ice cream (but please keep this to yourself). We all go through lapses in motivation. So how do you get back on track—or better yet, *stay* on track?

Step 6: Just Do Your Best Every Single Day, but Make Sure It's Your Absolute, Honest Best

Let's say that you go to the gym on Monday and do 12 reps of biceps curls with 30-pound dumbbells. Then you hit the treadmill, and 30 minutes of cardio fly by. You're psyched, you feel strong, and you know that you could take on The Rock if you met him in a dark alley. You leave the gym feeling as if you've had the workout of your life and go home happy, fulfilled, and "in the zone." Yet a few days later, you do the same biceps curls and can barely get through ten reps with the same weight. You start wondering, *What's going on? Why was I so strong on Monday?* Believe me when I tell you that this happens to everyone. It's virtually impossible to maintain the same strength and energy levels 365 days a year.

Here's where doing your honest best comes into play. When you got to that tenth rep, was it really the last rep you could muster with proper form, or did you quit early because you really wanted to get home and watch *The Bachelor?* Did you have another two reps in you? One more? Be honest with yourself—no one but you will lose if you aren't telling yourself your own truth. If you conclude that the tenth rep was really the last one you could do that day, then pat yourself on the back and be proud that you gave it all you had.

But if, as you drove home, you realized that you didn't do your best, don't beat yourself up and start feeling like you're a failure. That won't help your progress. Don't judge yourself so harshly—just make a mental note and turn up the fire tomorrow.

Step 7: Refocus Your Goals

When you're really lacking the motivation to stay on this program, it might be time to refocus your goals. First, remind yourself why you set these goals in the first place. Remember how you were—and still are—100 percent committed to making your goal a reality. When your commitment starts to weaken, look at what you wrote down. Envision what you'll look like when you achieve each goal. And think about how good you'll feel both physically and mentally when you're able to check off each goal and write "Accomplished" next to it. That should get you motivated again.

Step 8: Remember a Simple Equation: Results = Motivation

I'll let you in on a big secret: The ultimate penicillin to the anti-motivation virus is results. If you stick with your program long enough, you'll be excited by the changes you see and feel. There's something very motivating about having a healthier, happier life loaded with the increased self-esteem that comes from having a body you love.

Okay, enough talk. It's time to get to work.

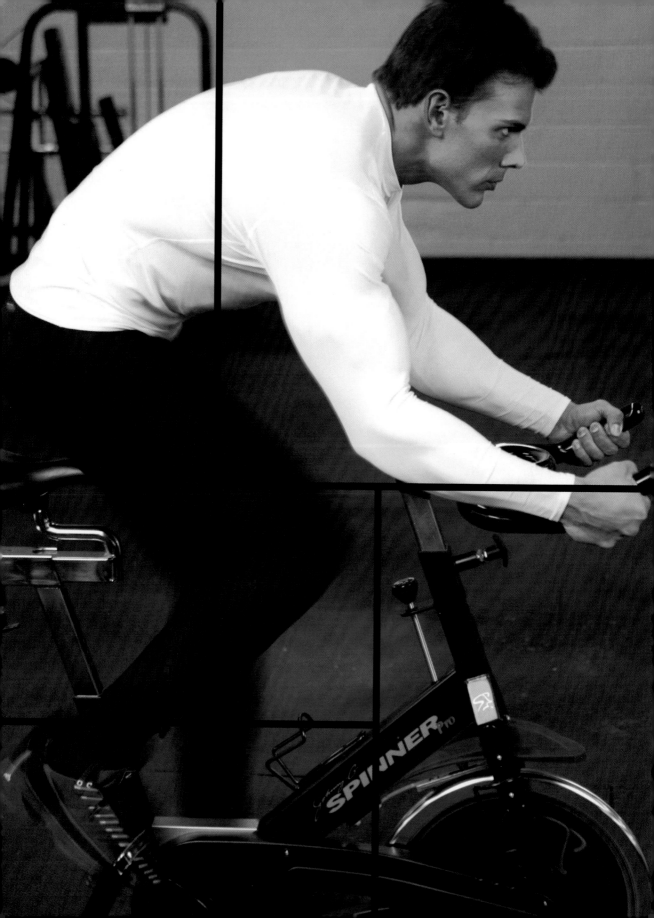

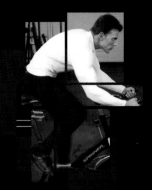

CHAPTER 5

THE IMPORTANCE OF STRETCHING AND CARDIO

Before we start melting away that fat, it's important for you to know something—I insist that every one of my clients include a stretching regime in their daily exercise routine. Stretching reduces and relieves stress, which can interfere with your sleep patterns, disrupt your diet, and weaken your immune system. And we all know by now that minimizing psychological stress is key to living a healthier life.

Stretching also reduces the physical stress you'll be putting on your muscles when you work out. Tight muscles are tense muscles, and muscle tension saps your body of energy. By alleviating muscle tightness, stretching reduces this tension. By the way, stretching your muscles also promotes muscle *growth*. This means that stretching can actually make the weight-training portion of your workout more productive, by accelerating and increasing your gains in strength and size. Finally, stretching can help reduce the soreness that normally follows when you push your body beyond its limits.

By far, the most important reason to stretch before exercising is to prevent injuries. When you stretch out thoroughly before a workout, you're much less likely to hurt yourself. I can't imagine going into the gym cold and doing even a single set of chin-ups without stretching. You have to properly prepare your body for the exertion you plan to put it through. If you don't stretch before working out, it's just a matter of time before you're going to injure yourself.

How to Begin Stretching

Before you begin *any* workout, you need to get your blood circulating and your muscles warm (even before you stretch). This can be accomplished by 5–10 minutes of cardiovascular exercise at low intensity. You can use a stationary bike, treadmill, rowing machine, elliptical trainer, or step machine; or you can slowly jog or do some simple jumping jacks. Keep in mind that this is your *warm-up,* or a way to prevent cold muscles from tearing. You won't be doing this to burn fat or exhaust yourself. I just want you to do this for 5 minutes, which will warm your muscles and speed up blood circulation. *Do not* go to the max because you could strain something. Remember that your body is still cold, and it needs this time to get into training mode.

Please always stretch carefully. I can't stress enough how important it is to keep these warm-up stretches light. I've seen a number of injuries occur when people come into the gym completely cold and start doing elaborate and difficult stretches. Careless stretching is just as likely to cause injury as working out without stretching or warming up first.

You have to listen closely to your body as you stretch. Move *slowly* through the exercise, and never bounce. *Feel* the stretch—feel your muscles relaxing, loosening, and lengthening as you do the movement. Gradually increase your range of motion with each rep. If you're stretching correctly, you should feel totally primed for the rest of your workout by the time you've finished. In fact, you'll be raring to go.

Let's begin with the simple stretches below. (Remember, you're not auditioning for the New York City Ballet—it's just you and me here.)

Stretching Guidelines

1. Stretch for 5 minutes.

2. Hold each stretch for 15–30 seconds.

3. Stretch until the muscle feels tight—never stretch until you feel pain.

4. Stretch slowly and don't bounce.

5. Stretch your entire body.

Standing Calf Stretch

Find a step or block of wood and place the balls of both feet on the step. Make sure you have something to grab onto to support your body. Step up as far as you can go on the balls of your feet, and then slowly lower your heels. Hold that lower position for 15–30 seconds, and then raise all the way back up on the balls of your feet. Repeat.

Lying Lower Back Stretch

Lie flat on the floor. Raise both knees, and place your hands just above your knees. Pull your knees toward your shoulders while raising your upper back off the floor.

Seated Hamstring Stretch

Sit on the floor with your legs straight out. Reach toward or past your toes (with your arms straight out), or bring your torso as far toward your feet as you can.

Chest
Stretch

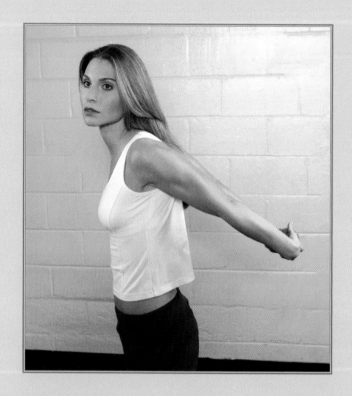

Back
Stretch

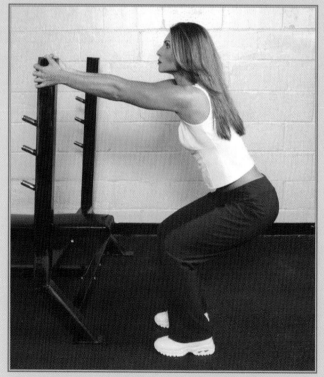

Chest Stretch

From a standing position, extend your arms straight behind you and interlock your fingers. Try to slowly turn your elbows in while straightening and lifting your arms as high as you can. Feel the stretch as you hold for 5–10 seconds, then relax and repeat.

Back Stretch

With feet shoulder-width apart, stand facing a heavy and stable gym machine that's at least as high as your shoulders. Firmly grasp the machine with both hands at shoulder height. Without moving your hands, slowly drop into a squatting position and lean back so that your arms are fully extended and supporting much of your body weight. Pull straight back and feel the stretch on both sides of your back as you hold for 5–10 seconds. Then shift your weight to the right, intensifying the stretch on your left side, and hold for 5–10 seconds. Next, shift your weight to the left, intensifying the stretch on your right side, and hold for 5–10 seconds. Stand back up, relax, and repeat.

Shoulder Stretch

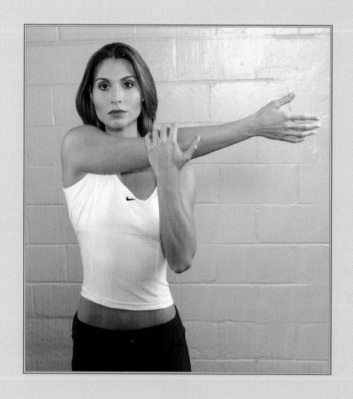

Quadriceps Stretch

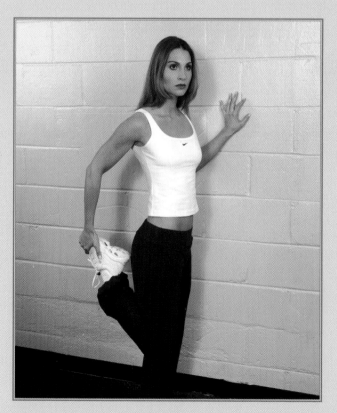

Shoulder Stretch

Stand with your knees slightly bent and your feet shoulder-width apart. Extend your left arm straight out to your side. With your right hand, reach out and grasp your left elbow. Keeping the rest of your body—particularly your hips and shoulders—motionless, pull your left arm across your body toward your right shoulder as far as you can. Feel the stretch as you hold for 5–10 seconds, then relax and repeat. Switch arms and repeat the exercise with your right arm.

Quadriceps Stretch

Stand next to a wall or sturdy machine with your knees slightly bent and your legs shoulder-width apart. Tilt your hips forward slightly. With your right hand, brace yourself against the wall or machine. Lift your left leg behind you, curling it up so that your foot approaches your butt. Grasp the top of your left foot in your left hand and slowly pull your foot towards your butt. Feel the stretch as you hold for 5–10 seconds. Return your left leg to the starting position, rest, and repeat. Then brace yourself with your left arm, and repeat the stretch with your right leg.

Hamstring
Stretch

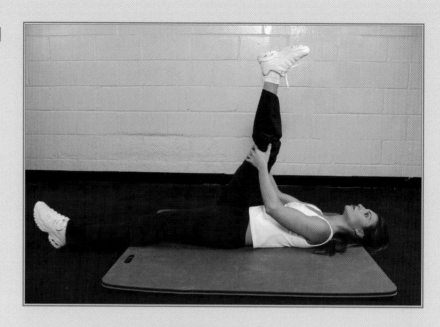

Calf
Stretch

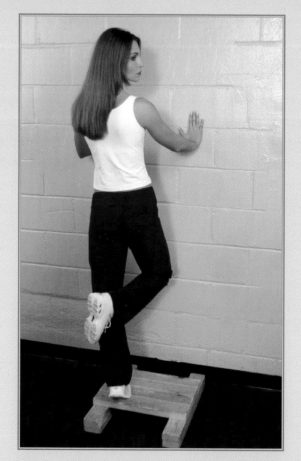

Hamstring Stretch

Lie flat on your back on the floor with your legs straight out in front of you. Keeping your right leg flat on the floor, lift your left leg up vertically so that it forms a 90-degree angle with your torso. Keep your lower back flat on the floor. Grasp your left leg behind the knee with both hands and slowly pull your leg down toward your torso. Feel the stretch as you hold for 5–10 seconds. Return your left leg to the starting position, rest, and repeat. Then switch legs and repeat the stretch with your right leg.

Calf Stretch

You'll need a step that's 4 or more inches high for this stretch (an actual step, a wooden block, a few stacked plates, or the foot-plate of a standing-calf machine or other machine with an elevated, horizontal foot-plate will do). Plant the balls of both feet on the step closer than shoulder-width apart and use both arms to brace yourself against the machine or a wall. Lift your right foot back behind you so that you're balancing on your left leg. Slowly lower your left heel down below the step as far as you can. Feel the stretch as you hold for 5–10 seconds. Then press back up, relax, and repeat. Switch feet and repeat the exercise with your right foot.

Congratulations. Now you're warmed up and ready to do some cardio!

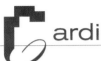ardiovascular Exercise

Welcome to the cardio section of *The TRUTH*. I know that a lot of you will want to cruise right past this section because you're thinking, *Man, I'm so sick of stupid cardio! It's not that important anyway. I'll just put on some muscle and lose weight that way.* Wrong! I wish that I could tell you it's okay to skip the cardio, but it's completely necessary.

I also hate to tell you that walking out your front door and getting into your car doesn't exactly qualify as cardiovascular exercise. I once had a consultation with a woman who told me that she didn't need me to put any cardio into her program because she usually parked two blocks away from her job. "That's more than enough cardio for the average person," she informed me, adding, "I also hate to sweat." I was speechless because she was totally serious!

There's no way around it: Cardio, diet, and weight training are a triple threat when it comes to making your waistline smaller and creating that healthy physique you desire. To break it down, diet (which we'll discuss in a later chapter) will help you lose body fat; weight training will build muscle; and cardiovascular exercise will chisel that muscle and control your weight while keeping your heart healthy. Let's use baseball as an analogy: To play the game, you need a ball, a bat, and a glove—if you're missing any one of these three items, you can't play baseball. The same thing applies to getting in shape: If cardio's missing from your program, you're going to fail at the game of life.

Cardiovascular disease is the number-one cause of death in the United States, and it's an equal-opportunity killer. According to statistics release by the American Heart Association, at least one out of every four Americans suffers from some sort of heart disease, and almost half of all deaths in the U.S. result from CVD. These statistics are staggering.

To me, it's a no-brainer: You need to sweat to survive. So let's get ready to move.

Finding Your Resting Heart Rate

I'm sure that every time you've picked up a fitness magazine or book, you've seen the words *resting heart rate (RHR)*. So what is that? Very simply, it's the number of times your heart beats per minute when your body is at rest. You measure your RHR by taking your pulse, and it's most accurately measured when you first wake up in the morning. Another option is to find a peaceful place, lie down, and remain still for 20 minutes, and then take your RHR. Your body needs to be in a total state of relaxation.

You may be wondering what your resting heart rate has to do with anything in *The TRUTH*. Well, it has *a lot* to do with the cardio part of the program. By knowing your RHR, you can gauge your workouts more efficiently and measure your improvements more precisely. It can also tell you if you've recovered fully from your training session and when (or if) you should proceed with your session. Knowing your RHR is crucial to making progress during your cardiovascular exercise program. (And keep in mind that as your RHR decreases, your fitness level will typically improve.)

How Do You Measure Your RHR?

You'll need to get a watch with a second hand. Now take the first two fingers on your hand and place them on your neck at the side of your throat. Press your fingers gently against the area. When you find your pulse, count the number of beats you feel within a one-minute time period. This will give you your RHR.

If you have a problem finding your pulse in your neck, try your wrist. Place the tips of your middle and index fingers on the inside of your wrist, in line with the thumb. Press down lightly and count the number of beats you feel within a one-minute time period to determine your RHR.

Your resting heart rate will indicate your basic fitness level. The average RHR for a man is 70 beats per minute (bpm), and for a woman it's 75 bpm. The better physical condition you're in, the less effort and fewer beats per minute it takes your heart to pump blood to your body at rest. Many people who work out consistently have a heart rate in the 50–60 bpm range. Extremely fit people and world-class athletes have a RHR in the 30–40 bpm ranges. But it's a good idea to be in the 70–90 bpm range when you're starting out.

If you find that your RHR is always high, even if you're exercising on a consistent basis, then you should seek the help of a doctor immediately. It could mean that you have a health problem or your training routine is too intense.

Heart-Rate Zones

We've already discussed the importance of knowing your RHR. The same thing applies to your heart rate, or the number of times per minute the heart contracts. A zone is a range of heartbeats, so your maximum heart rate (MHR) is the maximum amount of beats your heart pumps in a minute. When training on a cardiovascular exercise program, it's important to train at the correct intensity level. Perhaps you've asked yourself: *Should I go faster or slower? How do I know if I'm training hard enough? How do I know if I'm overtraining?* Well, that's where heart-rate zone training comes in. By following the simple equation below, you can find the correct zone to train in:

MHR for women = 226 – your age
MHR for men = 220 – your age

For example, if you're a 30-year-old man, the equation would be: 220 – 30 = 190.

The equation for figuring your target heart-rate range is: MHR x 0.55 (55%) to MHR x 0.90 (90%). Or, if we use the example above: 190 x .55 to 190 x .90 = 104.5 to 171. In other words, this man's target heart rate would be between 104.5 bpm and 171 bpm.

You should always stay within your target heart range—don't exceed your maximum heart rate. The best range for beginners is to stay within 55–60% of your maximum heart rate. Training in this zone will strengthen your most important muscle, the heart, and help you reduce cholesterol and blood pressure. You won't be able to increase your endurance and strength training at his rate, but you'll definitely reduce fat and become healthier. (For more advanced cardio trainers, I recommend performing your warm-up and cool-down in this zone. A slow bike ride or a brisk walk would help you obtain this range.)

If you want to burn fat, you need to be within 60–70% of your maximum heart rate. This is also known as the weight-management zone. Keep in mind the following:

- Working out at 70–80% of your maximum heart rate will help you improve your endurance, plus improve function of your lungs, heart, and respiratory rate.

- Working out at 80–90%* is a big step further; if you're training at this level, you'll have improved endurance and increased speed. You should only train in this range under supervision.

*Caution:** Exercising at 90% of your maximum heart rate is in the *anaerobic* range, which should only be done in short bursts. This range is so intense that your cardiovascular system can't get oxygen to the muscles. Professional athletes and Olympic runners usually perform in this range to increase speed or endurance. It's commonly used in interval training routines to help athletic performance—in other words, a person might do 2 minutes in this range to increase their heart rate. The threat of an injury is very real in this range: You can easily pull a hamstring, calf muscle, or worse training at this level.

For those of you who aren't so great at math, just take a look at this chart.

AGE	50% MHR	60% MHR	70% MHR	80% MHR
18–25	99	119	139	159
26–30	95	115	134	153
31–36	93	112	130	149
37–42	90	108	126	144
42–50	86	103	121	138
51–58	83	99	116	133
59–65	79	95	110	126
65+	76	91	106	121

(**Note:** Always wear a heart monitor during cardiovascular exercise so that you can monitor your heart rate at all times.)

Getting Started:
The Five Phases of Cardio Training

Here's how the cardio program breaks down:

1.   Warm-up
2.   Stretching
3.   Cardio activity
4.   Cool-down
5.   Stretching

Now allow me to outline the plan in detail.

Phase 1: The Warm-Up

Once again, I'd like to say that one of the biggest mistakes I see is people not warming up before they exercise. I always see people stretching as soon as they arrive at the gym. *I don't want you to do this.* You should never stretch when your muscles are cold because you could strain or tear the muscle—first you need to warm up your body and get the blood circulating. In order for you to do this, I'd like you to do a low-intensity cardio warm-up (walk, bike, treadmill, jumping jacks) at 50–60% of your maximum heart rate.

Phase 2: Stretching

If you aren't stretching before your cardio workouts, you aren't getting the most out of your program. It's like putting junkyard tires on a brand-new Ferrari: The car will still drive, but it will never reach its peak performance. See the beginning of the chapter to remind yourself of the stretches and why it's important to do them. Also, please practice correct form.

Phase 3: Cardio Activity

There are 4 levels of cardio, which are explained in detail at the end of the chapter.

Phase 4: Cardio Cool-Downs
(Read this or Frank will be mad at you!)

I know that after a long workout (or even a short one), the need to just get in that shower or drink a jug of water is strong. But do me a favor and give yourself a few more minutes to cool down before you leave the gym—5 minutes is all I ask of you.

A cool-down after cardio is extremely beneficial mentally and physically. Once you've completed your session of cardio, don't stop abruptly. You should take that time to physically recover and mentally unwind. You want to ease yourself back to normal and give your heart a chance to return to its resting rate without shocking it. It's a great thing to wait until your regular breathing pattern returns before you jump off that bike or treadmill. You don't want you heart to have to work overtime to return to normal—instead, cool it down.

Walk or bike slowly. Take time to reflect on what you've accomplished. You should mentally clear your head and think positive thoughts, praise yourself for accomplishing that half hour or hour of cardio. It's so important to finish your session with a clear and optimistic mind—if you believe that cardio activity is a positive experience, you'll want to do more. If you get off that bike with a negative feeling, however, every time you have to do your cardio you'll think, *Ugh, not this horror again!* The cool-down and the positive thoughts will remind you why you're here.

Phase 5: Stretching (Yes, Again)

We've already discussed the positive effect that stretching has on the body mentally and physically, but why should we stretch *after* our cardio session? For the same reasons that we stretch before we start cardio: to enhance our muscles' strength and flexibility.

Go ahead and do some of the simple stretches I outlined at the beginning of the chapter. You don't have to do all of them—just do a few to keep the cool-down working. Keep it very simple and brief.

The Four Levels of Cardio Training

Level 1

Let's get moving . . . gently. To begin, you'll be training at 50–60% of your maximum heart rate. A warm-up isn't necessary at this point because you're training at such a low heart rate (but you can do it if you want to); however, you should definitely stretch for 5 minutes after your workout. After you've finished this 30-day program, then you'll really kick into cardio-training.

The Workout

(Target 50–60% of your MHR)

1. Warm-up: 5 minutes
2. Stretching: 5 minutes
3. Cardio activity: See chart
4. Cool-down: 5 minutes
5. Stretching: 5 minutes

Once you've completed the first 30 days of the program, you should be feeling much better mentally and physically. When was the last time you walked for 30 minutes straight? I'm betting it's been a while. So take a couple of seconds and congratulate yourself—you're on the road to a new you, and you just got over the first obstacle! Do you remember what the first obstacle was some 30 days ago? It was getting started. Well, you not only started, but you finished what you set out to do. That's awesome! If you could do this, then you can accomplish anything, right? I know you can, so let's go to the next step.

Level 1 Cardio Program

WEEK 1	WEEK 2	WEEK 3	WEEK 4	WEEK 5 (if applicable)
Monday: Walk* 15 minutes	**Monday:** Walk 20 minutes	**Monday:** Walk 20 minutes	**Monday:** Walk 25 minutes	**Monday:** Walk 30 minutes
Wednesday: Walk 15 minutes	**Wednesday:** Walk 20 minutes	**Wednesday:** Walk 20 minutes	**Wednesday:** Walk 25 minutes	**Wednesday:** Walk 30 minutes
Friday: Walk 15 minutes	**Friday:** Walk 20 minutes	**Friday:** Walk 25 minutes	**Friday:** Walk 25 minutes	**Friday:** Rest
Weekend: Have fun, get out there and smell the roses	**Weekend:** Golf, bike, or do other fun activities	**Weekend:** Tennis, basketball, whatever you want to do for fun	**Weekend:** Play with your pet, etc.	**Weekend:** Fun, physical activity

*Walking can be substituted with biking

Level 2

Welcome to Level 2, which is designed for people who are active or who have been doing some sort of cardio exercise on a weekly basis. This program was designed to burn fat at a comfortable level of fitness. You have to walk before you can run. In other words, take your time with the program, enjoy it, and work at your own pace. Your goal is to lose weight, and to look and feel better. By following Level 2, you're going to accomplish just that—and much more. But remember one thing: *Don't overexert yourself at this point.* Why should you risk injury or a more serious consequence by trying to pedal or run at a faster speed?

Your goal at Level 2 is to burn fat, which is what you'll do working at 50–70% of your maximum heart rate. If you feel like 50% is too slow, feel free to pick up the pace. We talked about zones earlier in this chapter—do you know what the best fat-burning zone is? It's 60–70% of your MHR. That's exactly what you'll be targeting here, so relax and take your time. If you're feeling fatigued or in pain by doing cardio at 70% of your MHR, then slow down. You want to burn fat, not injure yourself.

Remember that you just removed yourself from your sofa a month ago—so take your time, build up your stamina, and get accustomed to doing cardio. Don't worry about running a marathon or biking the Tour de France. You should be excited about increasing your capacity from 30 to 40 minutes when just a few weeks ago you couldn't even do 20. These seemingly little victories are what keep you going mentally.

I know this is a 30-day program, but if you need extra time to get to the next level, please take it. If you take 60 days to complete this level, that's great. Please don't get discouraged if you're slow in progressing. Just remind yourself that you're doing cardio 3 days a week, you're burning fat, increasing your health, and creating a better mental and physical you. Your short-term goal is to finish this level and look and feel better.

Now, cardio shouldn't be boring and tedious—it should be fun. So what should you do? There are many activities to try, but I believe that the two most people can easily do are walking and biking. It's very easy to find a place to walk if you don't have time to go to the gym, and the same goes for riding a bike. I want you to get used to these two types of cardio because if you start doing the StairMaster every day but then can't make it to the gym for some reason, you won't do cardio that day. Conversely, everyone can find time to go for a walk, jog, run, or bike ride. I know that there are other types of cardio that you can do, but let's stick to the basics for now. You have to build a foundation in order to prepare your body for the next level.

The Workout

(You'll be training at 50–70% of your maximum heart rate)

1. Warm-up: 5 minutes at 50–60% MHR
2. Stretching: 3–5-minute full-body stretch
3. Cardio: Specified chart minimum of 30 minutes
4. Cool-down: 5 minutes
5. Stretching: 5 minutes

Level 2 Cardio Program

WEEK 1	WEEK 2	WEEK 3	WEEK 4 (and beyond)
Monday: 30 minutes biking or walking at 50–70% MHR	**Monday:** 35 minutes biking or walking at 50–70% MHR	**Monday:** 40 minutes biking or walking at 50–70% MHR	**Monday:** 40 minutes biking or walking at 50–70% MHR
Wednesday: 30 minutes biking or walking at 50–70% MHR	**Wednesday:** 35 minutes biking or walking at 50–70% MHR	**Wednesday:** 40 minutes biking or walking at 50–70% MHR	**Wednesday:** 40 minutes biking or walking at 50–70% MHR
Friday: 30 minutes biking or walking at 50–70% MHR	**Friday:** 35 minutes biking or walking at 50–70% MHR	**Friday:** 40 minutes biking or walking at 50–70% MHR	**Friday:** REST—you deserve it
Weekend: Fun, physical activity—Rollerblading, playing with a pet, etc.	**Weekend:** Golf, tennis, swimming, or any other fun physical activity	**Weekend:** Shopping, sightseeing, or other fun physical activity	**Weekend:** Yoga, kickboxing, etc.

Level 3

Welcome to Level 3! This program definitely isn't for beginners. You need to let your body get adjusted to a cardio program before you start this level because it's a 4-day-a-week program. Level 3 is all about increasing your duration while consistently staying at 60–70% of your maximum heart rate—the zone that I've found is the best for fat loss and weight management. (Go back and look over the zones if you need a little refresher.)

Now that you're more dedicated, Level 3 also mixes it up with other types of cardio. In the sample program below, I've given you a 30-day plan with a variety of different cardio activities. This program will also help you fight the boredom of doing the same thing day in and day out, and it will create new challenges for you. In addition, I've put together a plan that focuses on just the basics (walking, running, or biking) so that you can continue progressing if you're doing cardio outside of the gym.

If your goal is to lose body fat, tone up your physique, and get healthier, then this level will help you achieve those goals.

The Workout

(You'll be training at 60–70% of your MHR)

1. Warm-up: 5 minutes at 50–60% of your MHR
2. Stretching: 5-minute full-body stretch
3. Cardio: See chart
4. Cool-down: 5 minutes at 50–60% of your MHR
5. Stretching: 5-minute full-body stretch

In order to reach the target range of 60–70% of your MHR, I suggest fast walking, jogging, and biking. If you can't get your heart rate up by walking, then you need to pick up the pace and jog. If you have to jog to reach the target zone, then I strongly suggest that you bike 2 days a week and jog 2 days a week. I don't want you to get injured by running 4 days a week. I've seen many people's bodies break down from constant running—they can't absorb the constant wear and tear the body takes as a result from all that pounding. Remember, we're trying to lose fat, not run a race. Please switch up your routine and keep your body injury free.

Also, take as much time as you need in Level 3. You can do it for 2 months if you want before going to the next level. It's totally up to you. No matter what, you're still doing 4 days a week of cardiovascular exercise and creating a better body. And as we know by now, there aren't any drawbacks to that type of activity.

Level 3 Cardio Program

WEEK 1

Monday:
40 minutes fast walking, jogging, or biking at 60–70% MHR

Tuesday:
40 minutes fast walking, jogging, or biking at 60–70% MHR

Thursday:
40 minutes fast walking, jogging, or biking at 60–70% MHR

Friday:
40 minutes fast walking, jogging, or biking at 60–70% MHR

Weekend:
A fun physical activity—tennis, beach walk, Frisbee, etc.

WEEK 2

Monday:
40 minutes fast walking, jogging, or biking at 60–70% MHR

Tuesday:
40 minutes fast walking, jogging, or biking at 60–70% MHR

Thursday:
40 minutes fast walking, jogging, or biking at 60–70% MHR

Friday:
40 minutes fast walking, jogging, or biking at 60–70% MHR

Weekend:
Yoga, golf, racquetball, walk with a friend

WEEK 3

Monday:
45 minutes fast walking, jogging, or biking at 60–70% MHR

Tuesday:
45 minutes fast walking, jogging, or biking at 60–70% MHR

Thursday:
45 minutes fast walking, jogging, or biking at 60–70% MHR

Friday:
45 minutes fast walking, jogging, or biking at 60–70% MHR

Weekend:
Play with a pet, go bowling, attend an aerobics class, etc.

WEEK 4

Monday:
45 minutes fast walking, jogging, or biking at 60–70% MHR

Tuesday:
45 minutes fast walking, jogging, or biking at 60–70% MHR

Thursday:
45 minutes fast walking, jogging, or biking at 60–70% MHR

Friday:
45 minutes fast walking, jogging, or biking at 60–70% MHR

Weekend:
Swimming, surfing, or other fun physical activity—including sex!

WEEK 5
(if applicable)

Monday:
45 minutes fast walking, jogging, or biking at 60–70% MHR

Tuesday:
45 minutes fast walking, jogging, or biking at 60–70% MHR

Thursday:
Start new program or finish up the week on this program— it's up to you

Friday:
Start new program or finish up the week on this program

Weekend:
Fun physical activity

Here's a plan to add a little spice to your routine:

Variety Program Level 3

WEEK 1	WEEK 2	WEEK 3	WEEK 4	WEEK 5 (if applicable)
Monday: 40 minutes fast walking, jogging, or biking at 60–70% MHR	**Monday:** 40 minutes fast walking or jogging at 60–70% MHR	**Monday:** 45 minutes fast walking or jogging at 60–70% MHR	**Monday:** 45 minutes fast walking or jogging at 60–70% MHR	**Monday:** 45 minutes fast walking or jogging at 60–70% MHR
Tuesday: 40 minutes on an elliptical trainer at 60–70% MHR	**Tuesday:** 40 minutes on an elliptical trainer at 60–70% MHR	**Tuesday:** 45 minutes biking at 60–70% MHR	**Tuesday:** 45 minutes biking at 60–70% MHR	**Tuesday:** 45 minutes on an elliptical trainer at 60–70% MHR
Thursday: 40 minutes fast walking, jogging, or biking at 60–70% MHR	**Thursday:** 40 minutes on the StairMaster at 60–70% MHR	**Thursday:** 45 minutes fast walking or jogging at 60–70% MHR	**Thursday:** 45 minutes on the StairMaster at 60–70% MHR	**Thursday:** Start new program or finish up the week with this program
Friday: 40 minutes biking at 60–70% MHR	**Friday:** 40 minutes fast walking or jogging at 60–70% MHR	**Friday:** 45 minutes on an elliptical trainer at 60–70% MHR	**Friday:** 45 minutes fast walking or jogging at 60–70% MHR	**Friday/ Weekend:** Fun physical activities
Weekend: A fun physical activity	**Weekend:** A fun physical activity	**Weekend:** A fun physical activity	**Weekend:** A fun physical activity	

Notice that this particular program gives you a variety of different activities to do. You can substitute any of them except the walking/jogging, for I want you to continue to walk or jog twice a week. Don't let all of the other cardio machines take you away from the basics. When you're training on a StairMaster, elliptical trainer, or stationary bicycle, keep the intensity level relatively low. I don't want you to get hurt; I want you to burn fat. Focus on staying between 60–70% of your MHR—don't concern yourself with doing Level 12 on the bike or gliding up a hill on the elliptical trainer. You can set the machine to pinpoint a certain area of your lower body, but don't concern yourself with the intensity level. Stay low intensity, long duration (and between 60–70% MHR), and you'll reach your goals in no time. I promise.

Level 4

Welcome to Level 4! You're well on your way to the physique you've always wanted. By now each cardio session should be more challenging than the last, but you should still be giving 100% at all times. The only way that you can excel is by trying and pushing your body past those limits.

As an admitted training nut, I've tried all types of cardio at this level. I've done both low-intensity, long-duration (LILD) and high-intensity, short-duration (HISD) exercise—so which is better in conjunction with a weight-training program? My honest answer is that they're both beneficial. A lot of people get bored doing 40 minutes of cardio at a time, so they opt for a high-intensity 20-minute session. Some people's bodies get injured when following HISD—their muscles get pulled and strained when they push their bodies that far, so they like the slower pace of LILD. It all depends on what you enjoy doing.

I believe that if you're looking for a great way to improve your cardiovascular fitness, then your program should include a combination of both LILD and HISD. Anyone I train at Level 4 does a combo of the two. You'll see how it works in the sample programs below.

The Workout

(You'll be training between 50–80% of your MHR)

1. Warm-up: 5 minutes at 50–60% MHR
2. Stretching: 5-minute full-body stretch
3. Cardio: See chart
4. Cool-down: 5 minutes at 50–60% of MHR
5. Stretching: 5-minute full-body stretch

Make sure that you're fully warmed up before you start this program, as it's very easy to get injured running or biking at 80–90% of your MHR. Please take the time to follow the guidelines in this chapter. It's also important to wear a heart monitor when performing these exercises because you want to ensure that you're staying in the right range.

Level 4 Cardio Program

WEEK 1	WEEK 2	WEEK 3	WEEK 4
Monday: 45 minutes cardio activity of your choice at 60–70% MHR	**Monday:** 50 minutes cardio activity of your choice at 60–70% MHR	**Monday:** 55 minutes cardio activity of your choice at 60–70% MHR	**Monday:** 60 minutes cardio activity of your choice at 60–70% MHR
Tuesday: 45 minutes cardio activity of your choice at 60–70% MHR	**Tuesday:** 50 minutes cardio activity of your choice at 60–70% MHR	**Tuesday:** 55 minutes cardio activity of your choice at 60–70% MHR	**Tuesday:** 60 minutes cardio activity of your choice at 60–70% MHR
Thursday: 50 minutes cardio activity of your choice at 60–70% MHR	**Thursday:** 55 minutes cardio activity of your choice at 60–70% MHR	**Thursday:** 60 minutes cardio activity of your choice at 60–70% MHR	**Thursday:** 60 minutes cardio activity of your choice at 60–70% MHR
Friday: 45 minutes cardio activity of your choice at 60–70% MHR	**Friday:** 55 minutes cardio activity of your choice at 60–70% MHR	**Friday:** 60 minutes cardio activity of your choice at 60–70% MHR	**Friday:** 60 minutes cardio activity of your choice at 60–70% MHR
Weekend: Fun physical activity	**Weekend:** Fun physical activity	**Weekend:** Fun physical activity	**Weekend:** Fun physical activity

For the interval program, you'll be starting at 3 cycles of 3 minutes each. The first minute will be at 80–90% of your MHR (or running or biking at full speed) followed by 2 minutes of 60–70% of your MRH. When you complete the 21-minute program, you'll have performed 7 cycles. If you start progressing, increase the amount of cycles to 9.

This program can be done 4 days a week—and you can also follow the day-to-day schedule from the other Level 4 programs. I suggest that you switch up your cardio to do both the interval training and the long-duration programs.

Level 4 Interval Program

(Short-Duration, High-Intensity Cardio)

MONDAY, TUESDAY, THURSDAY, FRIDAY SCHEDULE

MINUTES	MAXIMUM HEART RANGE
Minute 1	80–90% MHR
Minute 2	60–70% MHR
Minute 3	60–70% MHR
Minute 4	80–90% MHR
Minute 5	60–70% MHR
Minute 6	60–70% MHR
Minute 7	80–90% MHR
Minute 8	60–70% MHR
Minute 9	60–70% MHR
Minute 10	80–90% MHR
Minute 11	60–70% MHR
Minute 12	60–70% MHR
Minute 13	80–90% MHR
Minute 14	60–70% MHR
Minute 15	60–70% MHR
Minute 16	80–90% MHR
Minute 17	60–70% MHR
Minute 18	60–70% MHR
Minute 19	80–90% MHR
Minute 20	60–70% MHR
Minute 21	60–70% MHR

It's not unheard of to do cardio more than 4 days a week, so if you strongly feel that it's not enough, you can do it more frequently. Just make sure that your body is recuperating and progressing in a positive manner before you add another day or two. If you choose to do cardio more than 4 days a week, then I'd primarily do low-intensity, long-duration cardio mixing in some sessions of short-duration, high-intensity cardio. I'd focus more on the long-duration cardio, because there's less wear and tear on the body. Your body won't be able to withstand the punishment of doing high-intensity cardio day in and day out.

Remember that your body needs rest and recuperation to repair itself from your daily workouts. You should also make sure you're eating enough calories to support the extra cardio you're doing. You don't want to start burning that hard-earned muscle you built.

Level 4 Long-Duration Program

WEEK 1	WEEK 2	WEEK 3	WEEK 4 (and beyond)
Monday: 60 minutes at 60–70% MHR	**Monday:** 21-minute interval program	**Monday:** 60 minutes at 60–70% MHR	**Monday:** 60 minutes at 60–70% MHR
Tuesday: 21-minute interval program	**Tuesday:** 60 minutes at 60–70% MHR	**Tuesday:** 21-minute interval program	**Tuesday:** 21-minute interval program
Thursday: 60 minutes at 60–70% MHR	**Thursday:** 21-minute interval program	**Thursday:** 60 minutes at 60–70% MHR	**Thursday:** 60 minutes at 60–70% MHR
Friday: 21-minute interval program	**Friday:** 60 minutes at 60–70% MHR	**Friday:** 21-minute interval program	**Friday:** 21-minute interval program
Weekend: Fun physical activity	**Weekend:** Fun physical activity	**Weekend:** Fun physical activity	

Here's an example of a five-day-a-week cardio plan:

Level 4 Five-Day-a-Week Cardio Plan

WEEK 1	WEEK 2	WEEK 3	WEEK 4
Monday: 60 minutes at 60–70% MHR	**Monday:** 60 minutes at 60–70% MHR	**Monday:** 60 minutes at 60–70% MHR	**Monday:** 60 minutes at 60–70% MHR
Tuesday: 60 minutes at 60–70% MHR	**Tuesday:** 60 minutes at 60–70% MHR	**Tuesday:** 60 minutes at 60–70% MHR	**Tuesday:** 60 minutes at 60–70% MHR
Wednesday: OFF	**Wednesday:** OFF	**Wednesday:** OFF	**Wednesday:** OFF
Thursday: 21-minute interval program	**Thursday:** 21-minute interval program	**Thursday:** 21-minute interval program	**Thursday:** 21-minute interval program
Friday: 60 minutes at 60–70% MHR	**Friday:** 60 minutes at 60–70% MHR	**Friday:** 60 minutes at 60–70% MHR	**Friday:** 60 minutes at 60–70% MHR
Saturday: OFF	**Saturday:** OFF	**Saturday:** OFF	**Saturday:** OFF
Sunday: 60 minutes at 60–70% MHR	**Sunday:** 60 minutes at 60–70% MHR	**Sunday:** 60 minutes at 60–70% MHR	**Sunday:** 60 minutes at 60–70% MHR

Stretch. Feel good. Take a deep breath. Hear me saying these words: "I'm really proud of you." And now it's time to pump some iron.

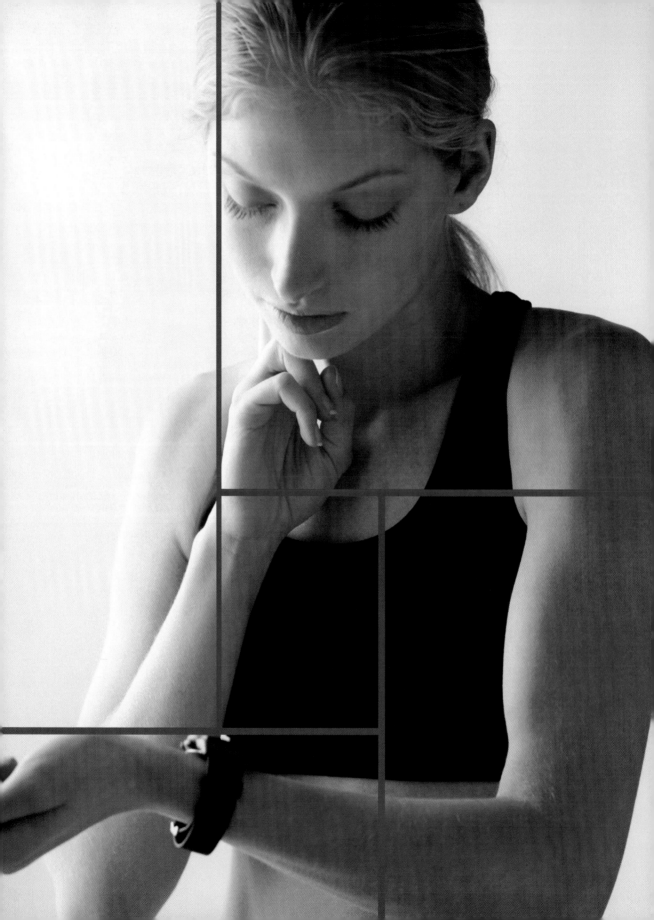

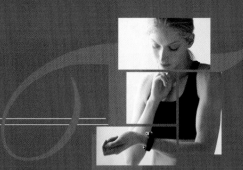

PART II
The Strength-Training Levels

Now that you've got the moves down, it's time to make a concrete plan for yourself. I know that many of you are thinking, *Frank, if I do <u>all</u> the exercises in Part II, I'll keel over!* Don't worry—I never expected you to do everything at once. Believe me, even *I* couldn't do them all at one time.

Actually, when you look through the levels, you'll discover that you're going to be doing far less than you ever imagined *and* getting more out of your workout than ever before.

So where should you begin? This handy little quiz should help determine what level you should be on. Please take a second and honestly answer the following questions:

1. In the last six months, has the only thing you've "picked up" been a restaurant check?

2. Does your idea of an "arm curl" entail moving a beverage to your lips?

3. Can your nine-year-old daughter/nephew/kid down the street beat you at arm wrestling?

4. On windy days, does your arm flap in the breeze?

5. *Bench press, squats, crunches*—are these foreign terms to you?

6. Do you have to dial 911 to have someone open a jar for you?

7. Were people wearing leg warmers and off-the-shoulder sweatshirts the last time you worked out?

If you answered yes to any of the above, it's time to begin at Level 1. However, if you feel that your fitness level is a little more advanced, then try starting at Level 2—but know that you can always go back to Level 1 if it's too much for you. *Please* don't jump ahead in levels, thinking that it's some sort of competition to work at a more advanced pace. Just like a home needs a foundation, I'd like you to work your way up the "level ladder" by building on your accomplishments.

If you're still confused, let me boil it down for you:

LEVEL 1 is a beginner's level, which has been designed for people who have never picked up a weight in their lives. You'll learn how to perform some basic movements, get the blood flowing, and wake up those muscles that haven't been used in a while. This is the ultimate novice's circuit training program, and it will yield great results while motivating you to get to the next level.

LEVEL 2 has been designed for people who lift occasionally or who have tried other beginner programs with mixed or absolutely no results. This program is a bit more advanced than Level 1 and allows you to really get to work on each body part.

LEVEL 3 is for intermediate weight trainers who have been on another program for too long or who need a new challenge to achieve even greater results. (You'll also graduate to this level after completing Levels 1 and 2.) Level 3 will add exciting secondary exercises that will put that extra polish on your new physique.

LEVEL 4 is an even more advanced routine for those who have graduated from the first 3 levels or for people who have been seriously training for years and really want to push it. Give me the same dedication and commitment that you've always brought to the gym, and I'll help you create the body of your dreams. I'll cover all of the advanced exercises that will refine your body and bring it to true greatness.

LEVEL 5—just when you're thinking I've pushed you to the limit, I'll go wild and introduce you to secrets I've never revealed before to keep your body at a maximum level. We'll also work on keeping workouts fresh, fun, and effective.

Remember that there are some common denominators for all the levels—including stretching, cardio, and the nutrition tips I'll tell you about in a later chapter.

It's time to select your level and go for it!

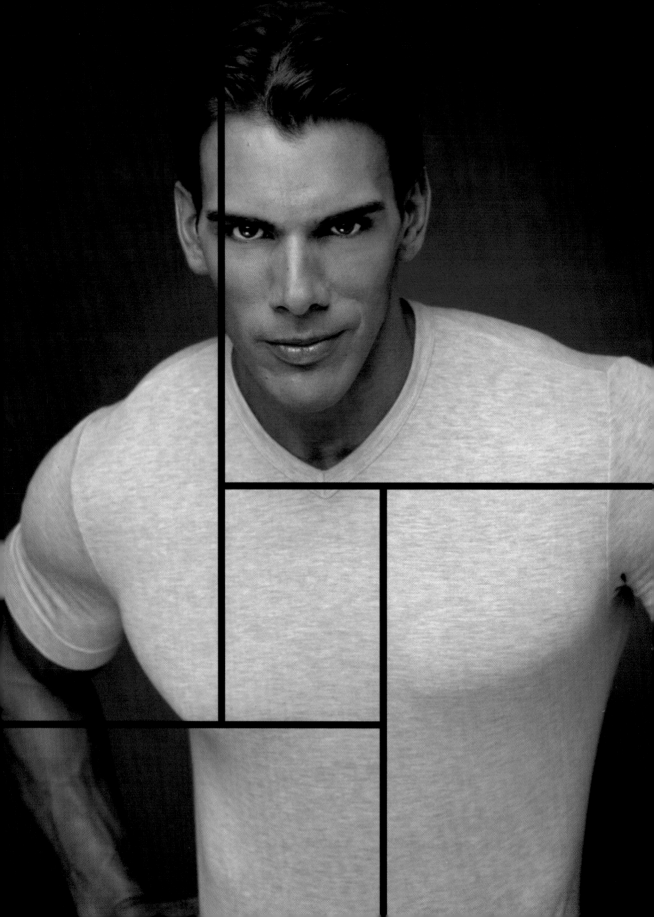

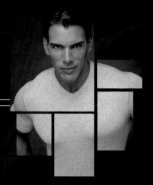

LEVEL 1

Welcome to Level 1! Remember, we're starting *today*. If you want to make positive physical and mental changes in your life, then there's no better time to begin than right now.

This program was designed for people who have access to a gym. I know that not all gyms are created equal, so feel free to substitute similar exercises if your gym is lacking a particular piece of equipment.

And keep in mind that you'll be combining cardio and weight work. (Please go back to Chapter 5 to recall which days you're "on" when it comes to sweating it off.) Each workout will take about an hour of your time, but it will be worth it.

Level 1 is perfect place for the newbie—in a nutshell, the program is 28 days long, but you'll only be working out for 12 of them. You'll exercise 3 days a week with at least 1 day off between each workout day. (Please, no need to thank me now—just send nice cards and letters!) And it's for men and women of all ages. Let's say that the last time you were in an actual gym was the sixth grade—this is your level. This is also a great level for senior citizens who want to improve their health. You're never too old to start weight training, and getting some cardio is an excellent way to stay in shape and remain vital. Cardiovascular activity helps maintain good circulation and keeps your heart pumping, while weight training benefits not only your muscles, but also your bones. That's true for people of any age.

However, I don't want you to think that this level is easy because it's strictly a no-nonsense program and the first step in a lifelong plan to feel and look better. (Remember that I advise you to check with your doctor before starting any exercise program.)

Now let's get to a quick round of "getting-started questions," which first-time clients often ask me:

"How sore am I going to be? I want to be able to drive my car and walk the dog on the days I exercise." Of course you can expect a minimal amount of discomfort—after all, when you work muscles that probably haven't seen much action in years, they're gonna get sore. You body will let you know that you've started an exercise program. But I promise that the soreness you feel should be mild, and your dog will get walked. I'm not the kind of trainer who'll put a beginner like you through such an intense workout that you're crippled with pain. I want you to feel ready to work out again in a day or so. We're going to stimulate sleeping muscle fibers, not fray them. I don't believe in "no pain, no gain."

"How is this weight-lifting program different from all of the other starter fitness programs out there?" Level 1 of The TRUTH program is different because not only will it get you in better shape, it will also get you ready for the next level.

There are many different short-term fitness programs out there, but The TRUTH is a *lifetime program* that carries you forward one level at a time. The first 28 days are crucial, for here you'll learn how to do almost every conceivable weight-training exercise. Level 1 will teach you how to work your muscles from many different angles, so you'll never do the same workout twice.

"Run this by me one more time: I'm only working out three days a week at first?" That's right—you'll be working out just three days a week for an hour, including cardio, and you can have the weekends off. You'll work out 12 out of 28 days, and you'll perform 12 different work-outs that work your entire body. Achieving symmetry is an important goal when you weight-train, and my routines are designed to build a healthy, symmetrical body.

If you've followed the regimen faithfully, you'll be in noticeably better shape after 28 days—that's the bottom line. You'll have more muscle tone, your clothes will fit better, and your cardiovascular capacity will be increased.

"How many exercises do I have to do?" You'll be doing 12 different total-body workouts. Remember that our goal is to build a symmetrically toned physique. So each workout consists of 8 weight-resistance exercises and 2 abdominal exercises for a total of 10 exercises.

"How do I pick the right weight to lift?" There's only one way to figure out how much weight you should be using for any particular exercise: trial and error. If you're doing the **Biceps curl–barbell** exercise and you can only curl the weight a couple of times, then the bar is obviously too heavy.

In Level 1, you should be doing 12 to 14 repetitions of an exercise for each set, so switch to a lighter weight and see if you can do 8 reps. Conversely, if the first weight you pick allows you to do more than 15 reps, go heavier for your next set.

"How long should I rest between sets?" In Level 1, you should rest for 90 seconds after each set. However, if you need a little more time when you're first starting out, go ahead and take it. Don't do another set until your normal breathing pattern has returned.

Be consistent in how much rest you take—don't take 1 minute here and 5 minutes there. Stay focused and alert. When you start Level 2, the rest interval between sets will be shorter because the shorter the rest interval, the more challenging the workout.

Another word of advice: It's very easy to get distracted in the gym—you can quickly get thrown off your game by chatting with your fellow fitness enthusiasts. Don't let it happen. There'll be plenty of time to talk after your workout. This hour in the gym is about *you*. Don't let distractions mess up your workout.

"What if this program is too easy? Should I increase the number of sets and reps that I do?" Absolutely not! There will be plenty of time for overachieving later. Right now you need to stick to the *exact* program and let your body get acclimated to the different exercises. This is the time to make sure that you're learning how to do each exercise with perfect form. You can seriously injure yourself if you try to accelerate too fast in an exercise program, especially when you're just learning how to do the exercises. Also, if you get hurt, your program will be interrupted before it gets off the ground—so give it time.

If you've spent a number of years being out of shape, what's the rush to achieve physical perfection all of a sudden? Rome wasn't built in a day, and you won't build up your muscles in a 24-hour period. Besides, there's no need to adjust the number of sets and reps you're doing in order to make the program more difficult. You already have complete control over how hard you're working because you're selecting the weight you lift—that's all the control you need in Level 1. You'll learn to intensify each exercise by changing multiple variables in the succeeding levels.

"I play tennis once a week. Does that count as a workout? Should I just work out two days a week to compensate?" Let's say Michael Jordan came to me and asked if playing an NBA game could get him out of one of the sessions. No way! I don't care if you're a professional baseball player who plays 7 games a week. This program is designed for 3 days a week, so it will only be effective if it's done 3 days a week. Tennis, golf, kayaking, and shooting hoops with your buddies are all worthwhile athletic endeavors, but they aren't part of your training program.

I'd encourage you to pursue as many athletic activities as possible to challenge your body in ways that it can't be challenged in the gym, as well as for your own enjoyment. But these kinds of pursuits aren't a substitute for the kind of training we'll do together. On the plus side, my program will actually improve your tennis game by making you leaner and stronger and increasing your cardiovascular capacity.

"What if I miss a day?" What? I don't think I heard you correctly. Miss a day? (Yes, I'm laughing hard right now.) You should *never* miss a day. When you start this program, you need to completely devote yourself to it, because it will only work if you give it 100%. Remember the saying "You only get out of something what you put into it."

If you miss a day because you didn't feel like working out, your car broke down, or you were worried about global warming, then you need to ask yourself, "Do I really want to change my life?" If your answer is yes, than you'll get off your lazy behind and go to the gym. Excuses aren't welcome here.

As a personal trainer, I've heard every excuse in the book. My favorite was this one: "I didn't know today was Tuesday." This guy worked in a bank—don't you think he knew what day it was? Of course he did—he just wasn't ready to give his fitness regimen his all.

I don't want to be a total hard-ass here: If you have a legitimate reason why you missed a workout, such as a death in the family or a serious illness, then you can work around it. After your missed day, continue to follow the workout schedule as planned, but add an additional week to your program. Yes, that's right—if you miss a day, add a week. You need to do the full program in order to move to the next level. Consistency is the key to success, so please don't miss any of the 12 workouts in the first 28 days.

"What if my gym doesn't have the equipment needed to do one of the exercises listed in Level 1?" I'm sure that there might be an exercise or two that you can't do because your gym doesn't have a particular piece of equipment. Don't worry about it. Just substitute another exercise from the list for that same muscle or muscle group. For example, if your gym doesn't have a crunch machine, substitute a crunch, knee tuck, or sit-up; or use a decline board instead of the crunch machine. You'll still be working your upper or upper/middle abs.

Monitoring Your Progress

There are really only three ways of monitoring your progress that matter: (1) Pay attention to how you feel; (2) take a look in the mirror; and (3) ask yourself if you're getting closer to your personal goals. If you feel better, like the way you look, and are closing in on your goals, then you're making excellent progress. If construction workers are whistling at you or your partner yells "Yowza!" when you get out of the shower, well, there you have it!

Of course there are a lot of other measures of success: weight or measurement changes; a decrease in body fat; and the ability to do longer cardio workouts, lift more weight, and do more reps. So in order to keep track of all of these things, you need to keep a training journal.

It's impossible to remember every exercise you've done, as well as how many reps you did and how much weight you lifted in each set, but you need to record that information on a daily basis. How are you going to know when you should increase the weight on a particular exercise if you don't remember how much weight you used?

I can't stress enough the importance of starting and maintaining a training journal. After all, your journal shows progress, and you should have significantly different numbers on Day 28 than on Day 1. A journal will tell you what your starting point was a week ago, along with which exercises you're excelling at and which ones are proving more difficult. The journal will also help you zero in on the times of day that you had your best workouts and when you didn't feel 100%. Recording all of these things is an important way to refine your training regimen.

Your training journal should include the following entry after each workout:

1. The Date

The first thing you should put in the journal is the date of each workout. Think of it this way: Each and every day you're recording your own personal quest.

2. Your Measurements

Before you start Level 1, use a cloth tape measure to measure your shoulders, chest, upper arms, waist, hips, thighs, and calves. For consistency, always measure each body part at its fullest point. (Your best bet is to have a friend measure you.) Then re-measure every part as you complete Levels 1–4 in the program. Once you've graduated to Level 5, you may want to re-measure every 3–6 months.

3. Your Weight

Pick a day and time when you're going to weigh yourself. Then do it at that same time every week because your body weight fluctuates throughout the day. For example, if you drink a bottle of water, you'll weigh a half pound more than you did before you drank it. That's why weighing yourself at the same time each week is important if you want to accurately record how your weight is changing. I recommend weighing yourself first thing in the morning—once a week—on an empty stomach. Don't get crazy and weigh yourself *every* morning because you'll want to flush the scale down the toilet (or worse!). And keep in mind that weight changes are only one measure of your progress. Just jump on the scale once a week *only,* and remember that this book does not advocate violence against scales!

4. Your Body-Fat Percentage

You can get your body-fat percentage tested at any local gym. They'll do what's called a "skin-caliper test," which isn't the most precise way to measure body fat, but it's accurate enough to give you an estimate of how much fat you're carrying around, and consistent enough for you to monitor your progress. The best body-fat test is one where you're submerged in water, but how often are most people going to trek down to the hospital for this test? The skin-caliper test is perfectly adequate. (You can also use a body-fat measuring scale, but I find them to be very inaccurate.)

5. Your Diet

Keep a complete list of everything you eat in a day and the times you eat it. This information is very important because you can use it to see how your body reacts to different foods. Then you can refine your diet to maximize weight loss and avoid wild swings in your energy level.

6. Your Cardio Routine

Write down exactly what you do for cardio—which exercise(s), how long you exercised, and at what intensity level.

7. Your Weight-Training Program

Every workout day, write the date at the top of a fresh page and then list all of the exercises you're doing that day. Record how much weight you use and how many reps you do for every exercise. You should also record how much time you rest between sets.

8. Subjective Workout Data

In addition to recording your sets, reps, and rest times, you should record how you feel when you're doing them. For example, if you're doing a particular exercise and you really feel great, write it down. Over time, this type of information will tell you what works and what doesn't.

You should also record how you feel mentally before and after your workout. Your mental state is just as important as your physical state. Starting a workout program is a lifestyle change, and any lifestyle adjustment is going to include a mental one as well. The goal of my program is to produce both positive physical and mental transformations. So write down info on your mind-set as you record your workouts in your journal.

Now that we've covered some of the basic pre-workout moves, it's time to hit the gym. Grab a bottle of water, and prepare to sweat! (Don't forget to refer back to Chapter 6 for detailed instructions on the exercises themselves.)

LEVEL 1 PROGRAM

PROGRAM DURATION: 28 days

WORKOUT FREQUENCY:
  3 days a week

WORKOUT TYPE: Full body

EXERCISES PER DAY: 10

SETS OF EACH EXERCISE: 2

REPETITION SCHEME: 12–15 reps
  per set

REST BETWEEN SETS: 90 seconds

DAILY WARM-UP

Cardio

  Cardio exercise of your choice,
  5 minutes at low intensity

Stretching

  Chest Stretch

  Back Stretch

  Shoulder Stretch

  Quadriceps Stretch

  Hamstring Stretch

  Calf Stretch

Day 1

Don't stress out—today's your first day, so it's going to take a little time to get adjusted to the gym. I know that at first it may seem overwhelming to find the right equipment, learn the exercises, maintain good form, try to find the correct starting weight, navigate the locker room, share equipment, snag a cardio machine, *and* remember to record everything in your training journal. Still, you need to block everything out and remember that you're in the gym for one reason: to find the true you. You can't let anything get you down. It's going to take time to get acclimated to the gym, so don't make any excuses.

If you can't do a standard push-up, do them with your knees on the floor. If you do an exercise wrong or can't immediately figure out how to do an exercise at all, that's okay, too. Everything probably won't come together right away—keep at it, and things will fall into place. Nothing worthwhile is easy. Believe me when I tell you that weight training isn't rocket science: *You will get the hang of it.*

Take a deep breath and have fun. Nobody said getting in shape shouldn't be enjoyable! So don't put undue pressure on yourself. You've taken the first step toward a fantastic new you. Stay positive and be patient.

Here is today's strength-training exercises (continue as directed on each following day):

CHEST: **Push-Up** (on your knees if a standard push-up is too difficult)
BACK: **One-Arm Row–Dumbbell**
SHOULDERS: **Shoulder Press–Machine**
TRICEPS: **Two-Arm Cable Push-Down–Straight Bar**
BICEPS: **Biceps Curl–Barbell**
ABS: **Crunch**
ABS: **Leg Raise–Vertical Bench**
UPPER LEGS: **Leg Extension–Machine**
UPPER LEGS: **Prone Hamstring Curl–Dumbbell**
CALVES: **Standing Calf Raise–Machine**

NOTE: Refer to Appendix: The Actual Exercises on pages 177 to 385 for a photo and description of each exercise.

Day 2

CHEST: **Fly–Dumbbell**
BACK: **Lat Pull-Down–Front**
SHOULDERS: **Side Raise–Dumbbell**
TRICEPS: **Skullcrushers–Barbell**
BICEPS: **Preacher Curl–Machine**
ABS: **Crunch**
ABS: **Knee Raise or Tuck–Flat Bench**
UPPER LEGS: **Leg Press–Machine**
UPPER LEGS: **Seated Hamstring Curl–Machine**
CALVES: **Seated Calf Raise–Machine**

Day 3

CHEST: **Incline Press–Barbell**
BACK: **Chin-Up**
SHOULDERS: **Front Military Press–Barbell**
TRICEPS: **Triceps Dip–Two Benches**
BICEPS: **Incline Biceps Curl**
ABS: **Seated Crunch–Rope**
ABS: **Reverse Crunch or Lying Leg Raise**
UPPER LEGS: **Squat–Smith Machine**
UPPER LEGS: **Standing Hamstring Curl–Machine**
CALVES: **Standing Calf Raise–Machine**

Day 4

CHEST: **Bench Press–Barbell**

BACK: **Row–Cable with V-Handle**

SHOULDERS: **Shoulder Press–Dumbbell**

TRICEPS: **Narrow-Grip Bench Press–Barbell**

BICEPS: **Biceps Curls–Cable with Straight Bar**

ABS: **Crunch–Machine**

ABS: **Leg Raise–Vertical Bench**

UPPER LEGS: **Hack Squat–Machine**

UPPER LEGS: **Stiff-Legged Dead Lift–Barbell**

CALVES: **Toe Raise–Machine**

Day 5

CHEST: **Incline Press–Dumbbell**

BACK: **Reverse-Grip Lat Pull-Down**

SHOULDERS: **Front Raise–Dumbbell**

TRICEPS: **Two-Arm Cable Pull-Down–Straight Bar**

BICEPS: **Preacher Curl–Barbell**

ABS: **Sit-Up–Decline Bench**

ABS: **Frog Kick**

UPPER LEGS: **Lunge–Barbell**

UPPER LEGS: **Prone Hamstring Curl–Dumbbell**

CALVES: **Seated Calf Raise–Machine**

Day 6

CHEST: **Incline Fly–Dumbbell**
BACK: **Bent-Over Row–Barbell**
SHOULDERS: **Upright Row–Barbell**
TRICEPS: **Kickback–Dumbbell**
BICEPS: **Biceps Curl–Dumbbell**
ABS: **Crunch–Decline Bench or Crunch Board**
ABS: **Hanging Leg Raise**
UPPER LEGS: **Step-Up–Barbell** (use a low platform: 12"–15")
UPPER LEGS: **Seated Hamstring Curl–Machine**
CALVES: **Toe Raise–Machine**

Day 7

CHEST: **Decline Press–Barbell**
BACK: **Reverse-Grip Row–Cable with Straight Bar**
SHOULDERS: **Front Military Press–Smith Machine**
TRICEPS: **Bent-Over Cable Triceps Extension–Straight Bar**
BICEPS: **Standing Hammer Curl–Dumbbell**
ABS: **Crunch**
ABS: **Hanging Reverse Crunch**
UPPER LEGS: **Squat–Barbell**
CALVES: **Donkey Calf Raise–Machine**

Day 8

CHEST: **Cable Crossover**
BACK: **Dead Lift–Barbell**
SHOULDERS: **Seated Bent-Over Raise–Dumbbell**
TRICEPS: **Triceps Push-Down–Rope**
BICEPS: **Biceps Curls–Cable with Straight Bar**
ABS: **Knee Tuck**
ABS: **Frog Kick**
UPPER LEGS: **Leg Press–Machine** (this time plant your feet high on the foot plate)
UPPER LEGS: **Leg Extension–Machine**
CALVES: **Seated Calf Raise–Machine**

Day 9

CHEST: **Dip–Parallel Bars**
BACK: **Reverse-Grip Lat Pull-Down**
SHOULDERS: **Arnold Press–Dumbbell**
TRICEPS: **One-Arm Cable Push-Down**
BICEPS: **Concentration Curl–Dumbbell**
ABS: **Kneeling Crunch–Rope**
ABS: **Knee Raise or Tuck–Flat Bench**
UPPER LEGS: **Squat–Machine**
UPPER LEGS: **Standing Hamstring Curl–Machine**
CALVES: **Standing Calf Raise–Machine**

Day 10

CHEST: **Bench Press–Dumbbell**
BACK: **Row–Machine**
SHOULDERS: **Rear Military Press–Barbell**
TRICEPS: **Overhead Triceps Extension–Dumbbell**
BICEPS: **Biceps Curls–Barbell** (this time, use the EZ Curl Bar)
ABS: **Crunch–Machine**
ABS: **Leg Raise–Vertical Bench**
UPPER LEGS: **Hack Squat–Machine**
UPPER LEGS: **Stiff-Legged Dead Lift–Barbell**
CALVES: **Donkey Calf Raise–Machine**

Day 11

CHEST: **Incline Press–Smith Machine**
BACK: **Row–Cable with Bar** (use a wide grip)
SHOULDERS: **Side Raise–Cable**
TRICEPS: **Triceps Dip–Machine**
BICEPS: **Seated Hammer Curl**
ABS: **Seated Crunch–Rope**
ABS: **Reverse Crunch or Lying Leg Raise**
UPPER LEGS: **Step-Up–Dumbbell**
UPPER LEGS: **Standing Hamstring Curl–Machine**
CALVES: **Toe Raise–Machine**

Day 12

CHEST: **Fly–Pec Deck**

BACK: **Dumbbell Pullover**

SHOULDERS: **Reverse Fly–Pec Deck**

TRICEPS: **One-Arm Cable Pull-Down**

BICEPS: **Concentration Curl–Cable**

ABS: **Sit-Up–Decline Bench**

ABS: **Reverse Crunch–Vertical Bench**

UPPER LEGS: **Lunge–Dumbbell**

UPPER LEGS: **Seated Hamstring Curl–Machine**

CALVES: **Donkey Calf Raise–Machine**

There you have it! It's not easy, but by the time you're on day 12, Level 1 will have become a part of your life. Just think about it: A few weeks ago you were lunging for the bag of chips, and now your thigh muscles are saying, "Time to come out of hibernation." This is major!

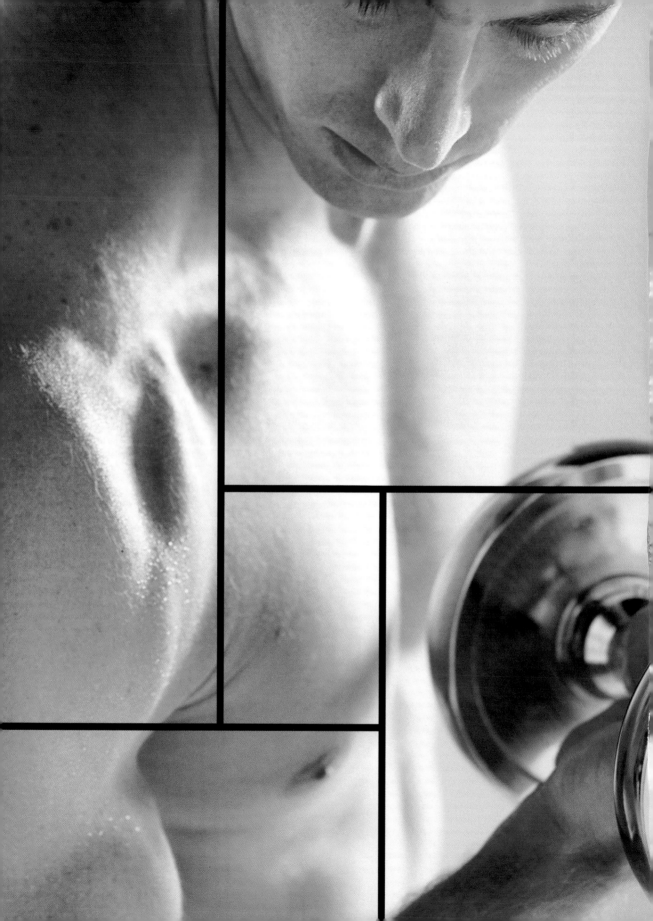

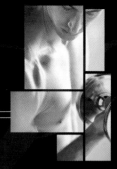

CHAPTER 7

LEVEL 2

Hopefully, you've successfully completed Level 1 and are feeling fantastic. See, it wasn't that tough, was it? Think back to 30 days ago and remember how you felt, how you looked, and how you felt about yourself—compare that to where you are now. Think of all the positive things that have happened to you because you took a chance and started this program.

Your body's probably looking better, your mind should be a lot clearer, and I bet that many people have commented favorably on your spiffed-up appearance, increased energy levels, and happier mood.

It's time to kick it up to Level 2. This is also the starting point for people whose prior exercise history has enabled them to skip over Level 1—that is, people who've trained with weights before and learned to perform the exercises correctly, but haven't been to the gym consistently. It's also a great next step for anyone who has been following a circuit-training regimen, or for people who have used other beginning programs but have failed to make any significant changes in their physiques.

It's All about You

You're in charge in Level 2. Yes, I've outlined the program for you—but instead of following a detailed regimen that I've dictated, you'll select individual exercises that *you* want to do. I've compiled a Master List of exercises that over the years I've found to be the most effective and rewarding for myself and for the hundreds of people I've trained. From that list, you can pick the exercises you want in order to tailor your workouts to meet your own unique needs.

Select exercises to tighten, tone, and shape your problem areas, then choose others to build new areas of your body. As your weight-training and cardiovascular work combine to melt extra fat off your body, you can choose exercises that will strengthen and build select muscle groups to subtly revise the overall shape and proportions of your body. Know that if you want to truly change your physique, then you need to keep changing your workouts. You need to constantly surprise and challenge your body.

The Master Plan

Level 2 is a personalized weight-training regimen that's designed to build an even, symmetrical physique while correcting your body's personal flaws. I've put together a master list of the most effective exercises you can do for stretching and for each of the body's eight main muscle groups: chest, back, shoulders, triceps, biceps, abs, upper legs (including butt), and calves.

Master Exercise List

(**Note:** Exercises in *italics* aren't pictured in the exercise description of this book. They're variations of the main exercise directly above them, and can be performed using form and motion that's nearly identical to that of the main exercise above.)

STRETCHING EXERCISES

Chest Stretch

Back Stretch

Shoulder Stretch

Quadriceps Stretch

Hamstring Stretch

Calf Stretch

CHEST EXERCISES

Primary

Bench Press–Barbell

Bench Press–Smith Machine

Bench Press–Dumbbell

Incline Press–Barbell

Incline Press–Smith Machine

Incline Press–Dumbbell

Decline Press–Barbell

Decline Press–Dumbbell

Dip–Parallel Bars

Secondary

Fly–Dumbbell

Fly–Cables with Bench

Fly–Pec Deck

Incline Fly–Dumbbell

Incline Fly–Cables

Decline Fly–Dumbbell

Cable Crossover

BACK EXERCISES

Primary

Bent-Over Row–Barbell

Bent Over Row–Dumbbell

One-Arm Row–Dumbbell

Dead-Lift–Barbell

Row–Cable with V-Handle

Row–Cable with Bar

Row–Machine

Row–T-bar

Chin-Up

Dumbbell Pullover

Secondary

Good Morning–Barbell

Lat Pull-Down–Front

Reverse-Grip Lat Pull-Down

Rear Lat Pull-Down

Stiff-Arm Lat Pull-Down

Shrug–Barbell

Shrug–Dumbbell

Seated Shrug–Dumbbell

Hyperextension–Machine

Reverse-Grip Row–Cable with Straight Bar

One-Arm Row–Cable

SHOULDER EXERCISES

Primary

Front Military Press–Barbell

Front Military Press–Smith Machine

Standing Front Military Press–Barbell

Standing Front Military Press–Smith Machine

Rear Military Press–Barbell

Standing Rear Military Press–Barbell

Standing Rear Military Press–Smith Machine

Shoulder Press–Dumbbell

Shoulder Press–Machine

Arnold Press–Dumbbell

Upright Row–Barbell

Upright Row–Cable

Secondary

Front Raise–Dumbbell

Front Raise–Barbell

Front Raise–Cable

Side Raise–Dumbbell

Side Raise–Cable

Side Raise–Machine

Standing Bent-Over Raise–Dumbbell

Bent-Over Raise–Cable

Seated Bent-Over Raise–Dumbbell

Reverse Fly–Pec Deck

TRICEPS EXERCISES

Primary

Narrow-Grip Bench Press–Barbell

Triceps Dip–Machine

Triceps Dip–Two Benches

Skullcrushers–Barbell

Overhead Triceps Extension–Dumbbell

Seated Overhead Triceps Extension–Dumbbell

Two-Arm Cable Push-Down–Straight Bar

One-Arm Cable Push-Down

Secondary

Kickback–Dumbbell

Kickback–Cable

Bent-Over Cable Triceps Extension–Straight Bar

Reverse Grip Cable Pull-Down–Straight Bar

One-Arm Triceps Pull-Down

Triceps Push-Down–Rope

BICEPS EXERCISES

Primary

Biceps Curl–Barbell

Biceps Curl–Cable with Straight Bar

Biceps Curl–Dumbbell

Incline Biceps Curl

One-Arm Biceps Curls–Cable

Secondary

Concentration Curl–Dumbbell

Concentration Curl–Cable

Preacher Curl–Machine

Preacher Curl–Barbell

Preacher Curl–Dumbbell

Standing Hammer Curl–Dumbbell

Seated Hammer Curl

Lying Biceps Curl–Cable

Standing Two-Hand Overhead Cable Curl

ABDOMINAL EXERCISES

Upper Abs

Sit-Up–Decline Bench

Crunch

Crunch–Decline Bench
   or Crunch Board

Upper/Lower Abs

Crunch–Machine

Kneeling Crunch–Rope

Seated Crunch–Rope

Knee Tuck

Lower Abs

Reverse Crunch or Lying Leg Raise

Hanging Reverse Crunch

Reverse Crunch–Vertical Bench

Leg Raise–Bench

Leg Raise–Vertical Bench

Hanging Leg Raise

Knee Raise or Tuck–Flat Bench

Frog Kick

Obliques

Twisting Crunch–Decline Bench
   or Crunch Board

Hanging Twisting Leg Raise

Seated Twist

UPPER-LEG EXERCISES

Primary

Squat–Barbell

Squat–Smith Machine

Half Squat

Squat–Machine

Front Squat–Barbell

Front Squat–Smith Machine

Hack Squat–Machine

Leg Press–Machine

Lunge–Barbell

Lunge–Dumbbell

Step-Up–Barbell

Step-Up–Dumbbell

Secondary

Leg Extension–Machine

Braced Squat

Lying Hamstring Curl–Machine

Prone Hamstring Curl–Dumbbell

Seated Hamstring Curl–Machine

Standing Hamstring Curl–Machine

Stiff-Legged Dead Lift–Barbell

Stiff-Legged Dead Lift–Dumbbell

CALF EXERCISES

Standing Calf Raise–Machine

Donkey Calf Raise–Machine

Seated Calf Raise–Machine

Toe Raise–Machine

Primary and Secondary Exercises

You'll notice that for most of the muscle groups, I've separated the exercise list into primary exercises and secondary exercises. What's the difference?

Primary exercises usually involve two or more joints and are often referred to as "compound movements." Think of them as exercises that work more than one body part—squats, for example, work your quadriceps, hamstrings, calves, butt, and lower back. Primary exercises involve both the largest muscles in a muscle group as well as the smaller, stabilizing muscles. These exercises will be the foundation of your workout because they utilize a great muscle mass and allow you to lift heavier weights than secondary exercises. They're excellent for building strength and lean muscle mass, and will help you improve your coordination, since they usually involve multiple joints and muscles and are crucial to building the foundation of your physique.

Secondary exercises generally involve only one joint in their movement. They're not great mass builders and won't help you get incredibly strong, but they're excellent for shaping and sculpting a muscle. When working a muscle group, do your secondary exercises after your primary exercises because the muscle you're working will be "pre-exhausted," or previously worked and fatigued.

Secondary exercises help promote muscle definition, which allows you to distinguish one muscle in a group from another. The next time you're at the gym, take a good look at somebody with a great pair of arms. Notice how their upper-arm muscles are separated so that you can easily distinguish the biceps from the triceps. In other words, you can see how secondary exercises will allow you to target specific areas of your body.

Let's focus on your triceps for a minute. Even though you'll be working them with **Bench presses** (a primary exercise for the chest), you can target the muscles better with **Triceps push-downs** (a secondary exercise). Primary and secondary exercises work synergistically—you can't build a shapely, muscular body without both of them. Of course, in order to have visibly well-defined body parts, you've got to keep your body fat down, which is where healthy eating and regular cardio work come in.

Calf and abdominal exercises are categorized differently: For calves, there are only four exercises, all of which could probably be considered secondary exercises because they're focused very tightly on the two muscles that make up the calf. So, where are the primary exercises for the calves? Think back to your workouts in Level 1. Did you ever find that your calves were tired *before* you did that day's calf exercise? I bet you did, because your calves were actually worked pretty hard by all of the primary exercises for upper legs, especially the different types of squats. By the time you get to the calf exercises, your calves are already half done. Great news!

This is also why you won't find forearm exercises listed in this book at all. Your forearms are used extensively when you work almost any muscle group in your upper body. They get a good workout whether you're working your chest, back, shoulders, biceps, or triceps. Unless you're a competitive bodybuilder, there's really no need to devote any time exclusively to developing your forearms.

As for abdominal exercises, all of the exercises listed here are very targeted. Instead of dividing ab exercises into primary and secondary, they've been grouped according to which area of your abs they focus on: upper, upper/middle, lower, or obliques.

For each body part, all you need to do is pick the exercises from the list that you feel will be the most beneficial in working your body's problem areas.

Level 2 Program

Level 2 is a 28-day program in which you'll train 3 days a week. I recommend Mondays, Wednesdays, and Fridays, since that's usually a good split for people who have full-time jobs or are stay-at-home parents. It allows you to have every other weekday off from the gym and leaves your weekends free. If you've just completed Level 1, you can stay on exactly the same weekly schedule—in fact, you'll be putting in the same amount of time as you did for Level 1 and getting even better results. I guarantee it!

Many people don't realize that whether you train 3 days a week or 5 doesn't really matter. What matters is what you do in those 3 days and how hard you work. Think in terms of the *quality* of your workouts, not the *quantity*. I've seen people who train 7 days a week and still look as if they've never seen the inside of a gym—don't be one of them! Then again, don't blame me if after you complete Level 2 you suddenly have the desire to go to the gym more often. That usually happens when people start seeing results.

For chest, back, shoulders, and upper legs, you'll perform one primary exercise and one secondary exercise; for biceps, triceps, and calves, you'll perform just one primary exercise. You can pick different primary and secondary exercises every time you repeat a muscle-group workout, or you can keep doing the same ones over and over. It's totally up to you. (The descriptions I supplied in Part II of this book also detail exactly which part or parts of a muscle group each exercise targets.)

You'll do 3 sets of each exercise, but the number of reps you do for each set will be variable. I recommend using a pyramid system for your reps for each exercise: Start off your first set with a lighter weight and progress to a heavier weight for each successive set. Your rep scheme should be 12-10-8 for your primary exercises. This means that you'll do 12 repetitions for the first set, 10 repetitions on the second set, and 8 repetitions on the third set. Your rep scheme will be different for the secondary exercises, which are focused more on greater reps than on heavy weight. The scheme will be 15-12-10.

Just as in Level 1, the only way to find the correct weight to lift for each exercise is through trial and error. For exercises you performed in Level 1, you can refer to your training journal to see what weight you lifted. For new exercises, you'll just have to choose a weight and lift it—if the weight is too heavy for you to do the prescribed number of repetitions, then switch to a lighter one. If the weight is so light that you do more than the prescribed number of reps without any trouble, then switch to a heavier one. It's that simple. The only way to find the right weight is by doing it.

How much weight should you add as you move from set to set on a particular exercise? You'll want to move up in small increments, and this will vary depending on the exercise. Let's say that you can easily bench-press 100 pounds 12 times. Try moving up in 10-pound increments for your subsequent sets. Your first set would be 12 reps at 100 pounds, your second set would be 10 reps at 110 pounds, and your last set would be 8 reps at 120 pounds. If you can do more than 8 or 10 reps on the second and third sets, add weight. If you can't do that many, then move the weight by smaller increments. The perfect weight is one that allows you to get the allotted reps in and no more.

You should be taking a 90-second break between primary exercises and 60 seconds between secondary exercises. If you need a little more time, please take it. Stay focused, because it's easy to get distracted in the gym and lose track of time. Remember that you're in the gym for one reason: to get in shape. Save the small talk and dating scene for after your workout. (Believe me, this will come into play more and more as you progress through this program— just call me Frank the Matchmaker!)

Moving on Up

You can go on to Level 3 when you've completed all 12 workouts in Level 2—and when you can honestly say that you've given 100% to every workout. You're only cheating or fooling yourself if you haven't. If you've just breezed through the Level 2 workouts without challenging yourself, then you're certain to have serious problems with Level 3. Conversely, you may have worked hard throughout all of Level 2 and still not be ready for Level 3. Everyone's different, and it's good to progress at your own speed. How do you know if you're not ready? Well, if you're having trouble with extreme soreness or fatigue after your workouts, then you shouldn't move on to Level 3. Give yourself another 2 weeks for your body to adapt to Level 2. After the 2 weeks, take stock of your progress and your program. If you feel ready, move on. But if you're still not ready, don't take it as a sign of failure. The bottom line is that even if you're not ready, you're still working out and bettering your physique. Isn't that the goal anyway?

LEVEL 2 PROGRAM

Exercise Schedule
Number of Sets and Reps, Rest Intervals, and Weight Schemes

PROGRAM DURATION: 28 days
WORKOUT FREQUENCY: 3 days a week

PRIMARY EXERCISES
3 sets of 12, 10, and 8 reps
90-second maximum rest between sets
Increase weight each set

SECONDARY EXERCISES
3 sets of 15, 12, and 10 reps
60-second maximum rest between sets
Increase weight each set

CALF EXERCISES
3 sets of 15, 12, and 10 reps
60-second maximum rest between sets
Increase weight each set

ABDOMINAL EXERCISES
3 sets of 15–20 reps
60-second maximum rest between sets

NOTE: Pick your primary and secondary exercises from the master list located on pages 83–85.

DAY 1	DAY 2	DAY 3	DAY 4	DAY 5	DAY 6	DAY 7
CHEST 1 primary 1 secondary **TRICEPS** 1 primary **BICEPS** 1 primary **ABS** 1 upper or upper/ middle abs 1 lower abs	OFF	**BACK** 1 primary 1 secondary **SHOULDERS** 1 primary 1 secondary **ABS** 1 upper or upper/ middle abs 1 lower abs	OFF	**UPPER LEGS** 1 primary 1 secondary **CALVES** 1 exercise **ABS** 1 upper or upper/ middle abs 1 lower abs	OFF	OFF

If you look at the Level 2: Sample Week, you can see just how easy it is to structure your workout.

Level 2: Sample Week

DAY 1	DAY 2	DAY 3

CHEST (6 sets)
Primary
   Bench Press–Barbell
   3 sets of 12, 10, and 8 reps
Secondary
   Fly–Dumbbell
   3 sets of 15, 12, and 10 reps
 	
TRICEPS (3 sets)
Primary
   Two-Arm Cable Push-
   Down–Straight Bar
   3 sets of 12, 10, and 8 reps
 	
BICEPS (3 sets)
   Biceps Curl–Barbell
   3 sets of 12, 10, and 8 reps
 	
ABS (6 sets)
Upper Abs
   Crunch
   3 sets of 15–20 reps
Lower Abs
   Leg Raise–Bench
   3 sets of 15–20 reps
	OFF	**BACK** (6 sets)
		Primary
		   Bent-Over Row–Barbell
		   3 sets of 12, 10, and 8 reps
		Secondary
		   Lat Pull-Down–Front
		   3 sets of 15, 12, and 10 reps
		
		SHOULDERS (6 sets)
		Primary
		   Shoulder Press–Dumbbell
		   3 sets of 12, 10, and 8 reps
		Secondary
		   Side Raise–Dumbbell
		   3 sets of 15, 12, and 10 reps
		
		ABDOMINALS (6 sets)
		Upper Abs
		   Sit-Up–Decline Bench
		   3 sets of 15–20 reps
		Lower Abs
		   Leg Raise–Bench
		   3 sets of 15–20 reps

Note: Don't forget your cardio!

DAY 4	DAY 5	DAY 6	DAY 7

OFF	**UPPER LEGS** (6 sets)
	Primary
	    Squat–Smith Machine
	    3 sets of 12, 10, and 8 reps
	Secondary
	    Standing Hamstring
	    Curl–Machine
	    3 sets of 15, 12, and 10 reps
	
	CALVES (3 sets)
	    Toe Raise–Machine
	    3 sets of 12, 10, and 8 reps
	
	ABS (6 sets)
	Upper/Middle Abs
	    Seated Crunch–Rope
	    3 sets of 15–20 reps
	Lower Abs
	    Knee Raise or Tuck–
	    Flat Bench
	    3 sets of 15–20 reps
		OFF	OFF

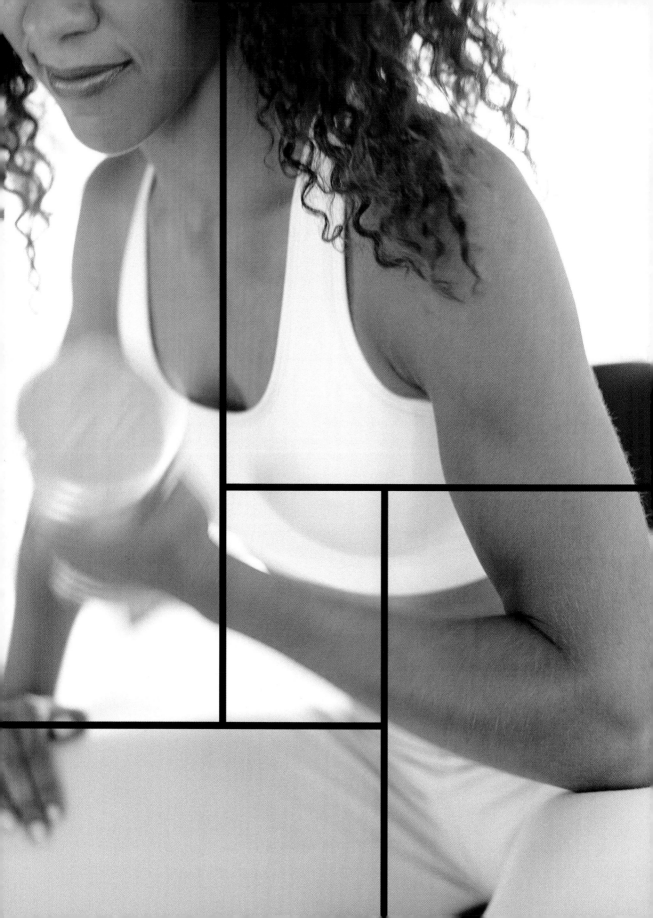

CHAPTER 8

LEVEL 3

Remember how good you were feeling after you completed Level 1? I bet it can't compare to how good you feel right now. In fact, perhaps *People* has called you for their "50 Sexiest People Alive" issue, wanting to put your story between George Clooney's and Catherine Zeta-Jones's.

Seriously, it's impossible to miss that your body is changing for the better. Everything is firmer, your body's proportions are changing, and you're really closing in on some of your short-term goals: an inch less here, a half inch more there; and a definite change in your weight.

Maybe you've bought some new clothes to fit your new shape, or maybe you've finally fit back into some of your old favorites. But the best thing of all is that your energy level during the day is through the roof, and you're sleeping better at night, too. There's no doubt about it: You feel terrific.

It's time to bring on Level 3. You're still in charge of your own plan. You'll continue to tailor your workouts to your particular needs and goals. You'll also select all of your exercises from the master exercise list featured in Chapter 7 (Level 2). You'll once again perform both primary and secondary exercises and select your abdominal exercises based on the specific areas you need to work. You'll also continue to perform multiple sets of each exercise in the pyramid format.

So what exactly is different in Level 3? Well, now we're kicking up the intensity level quite a bit. It's still a 28-day program, but now you'll work out 1 more day per week. You can still keep your weekends free if you like, but instead of working out on Mondays, Wednesdays, and Fridays, you'll be exercising on Thursdays as well. You'll still be working your abs 3 days a week with 2 exercises a day, but the workouts for all the rest of your muscle groups will gain an exercise. That's 2 exercises for calves; a primary *and* a secondary exercise for both biceps and triceps; and *2* primary exercises and a secondary for chest, back, shoulders, and upper legs.

Don't worry—I know you can handle it. Let's go!

LEVEL 3 PROGRAM

Exercise Schedule
Number of Sets and Reps, Rest Intervals, and Weight Schemes

PROGRAM DURATION: 28 days

WORKOUT FREQUENCY: 4 days a week

PRIMARY EXERCISES

3 sets of 12, 10, and 8 reps

90-second maximum rest between sets

Increase weight each set

SECONDARY EXERCISES

3 sets of 15, 12, and 10 reps

60-second maximum rest between sets

Increase weight each set

CALF EXERCISES

First Exercise: 3 sets of 12, 10, and 8 reps

Second Exercise: 3 sets of 15, 12, and 10 reps

60-second maximum rest between sets

Increase weight each set

ABDOMINAL EXERCISES

3 sets of 15–20 reps

60-second maximum rest between sets

NOTE: Pick your primary and secondary exercises from the master list located on pages 83–85.

DAY 1	DAY 2	DAY 3	DAY 4	DAY 5	DAY 6	DAY 7

BACK
2 primary
1 secondary
 	
ABS
1 upper or
  upper/middle
  abs
1 lower abs
	SHOULDERS
	2 primary
	1 secondary
	
	TRICEPS
	1 primary
	1 secondary
	
	ABS
	1 upper or
	  upper/middle
	  abs
	1 lower abs
		OFF	**UPPER LEGS**
			2 primary
			1 secondary
			
			CALVES
			2 exercises
				CHEST
				2 primary
				1 secondary
				
				BICEPS
				1 primary
				1 secondary
				
				ABS
				1 upper or
				  upper/middle
				  abs
				1 lower abs
					OFF	OFF

Level 3: Sample Week

DAY 1	DAY 2	DAY 3

BACK (9 sets)
Primary
   Bent-Over Row–Barbell
   3 sets of 12, 10, and 8 reps
   Row–Cable with V-Handle
   3 sets of 12, 10, and 8 reps
Secondary
   Lat Pull-Down–Front
   3 sets of 12, 10, and 8 reps
 	
ABS (6 sets)
Upper Abs
   Crunch
   3 sets of 15–20 reps
Lower Abs
   Knee Tuck
   3 sets of 15–20 reps
	SHOULDERS (9 sets)
	Primary
	   Front Military Press–Barbell
	   3 sets of 12, 10, and 8 reps
	   Shoulder Press–Dumbbell
	   3 sets of 12, 10, and 8 reps
	Secondary
	   Side Raise–Dumbbell
	   3 sets of 15, 12, and 10 reps
	
	TRICEPS (6 sets)
	Primary
	   Narrow-Grip Bench Press
	   3 sets of 12, 10, and 8 reps
	Secondary
	   Kickback–Dumbbell
	   3 sets of 15, 12, and 10 reps
	
	ABS (6 sets)
	Upper/Middle Abs
	   Crunch–Machine
	   3 sets of 15–20 reps
	Lower Abs
	   Leg Raise–Bench
	   3 sets of 15–20 reps
		OFF

DAY 4	DAY 5	DAY 6	DAY 7

UPPER LEGS (9 sets)
Primary
    Squat–Machine
    3 sets of 12, 10,
    and 8 reps
    Leg Press–Machine
    3 sets of 12, 10,
    and 8 reps
Secondary
    Prone Hamstring Curl–
    Dumbbell
    3 sets of 15, 12,
    and 10 reps
 	
CALVES (6 sets)
    Standing Calf Raise–
    Machine
    3 sets of 12, 10,
    and 8 reps
    Seated Calf Raise–
    Machine
    3 sets of 15, 12,
    and 10 reps
	CHEST (9 sets)
	Primary
	    Bench Press–Barbell
	    3 sets of 12, 10,
	    and 8 reps
	    Incline Press–Barbell
	    3 sets of 12, 10,
	    and 8 reps
	Secondary
	    Fly–Pec Deck
	    3 sets of 15, 12,
	    and 10 reps
	
	BICEPS (6 sets)
	Primary
	    Biceps Curls–Barbell
	    3 sets of 12, 10,
	    and 8 reps
	Secondary
	    Concentration Curl–
	    Dumbbell
	    3 sets of 15, 12,
	    and 10 reps
	
	ABS (6 sets)
	Upper Abs
	    Crunch–Decline Bench
	    or Crunch Board
	    3 sets of 15–20 reps
	Lower Abs
	    Hanging Leg Raise
	    3 sets of 15–20 reps
		OFF	OFF

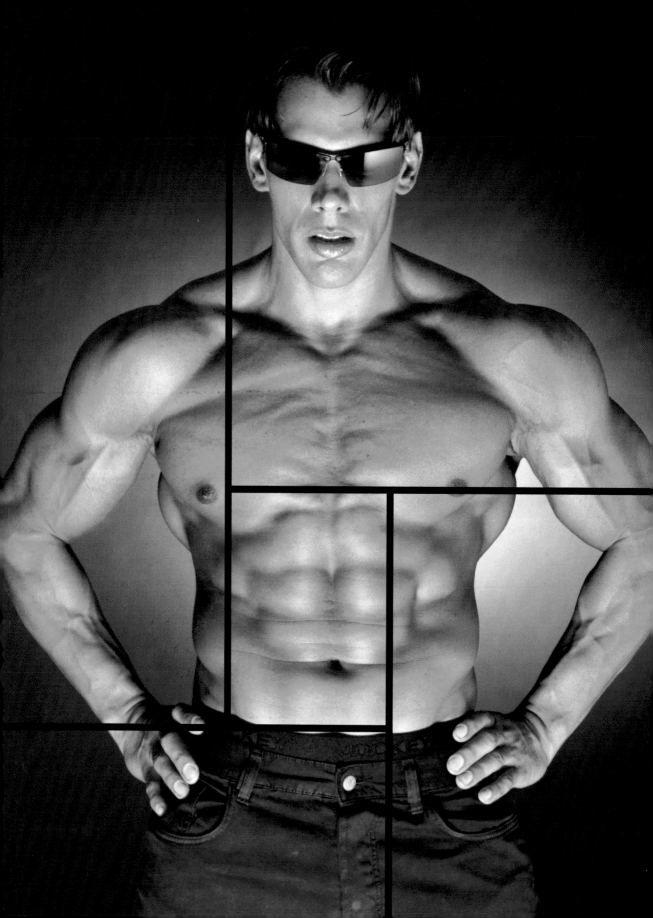

CHAPTER 9

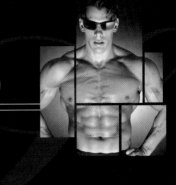

LEVEL 4

These days you look so good that when you flash store clerks your driver's license, they tell you, "Yeah, right—now show me your *real* I.D." When you see your own mother, she squints and says, "You remind me of someone who's about half the size of my child." Yes, it's hard to even pinpoint a resemblance between your old body and your new one . . . so it must be time to take it to the next level.

I'm sure you're completely familiar with the drill by now. In Level 4, you'll continue to select all of your exercises from the master exercise list featured in Chapter 7 (Level 2). And you'll still work out 4 days a week, so you can stick to the same weekly schedule. Yet, in other ways, your workouts will continue to intensify.

First, you'll be adding another secondary exercise to the workout for the largest of the major muscle groups. In other words, you'll do 2 primary and 2 secondary exercises for the chest, back, shoulders, and upper legs. We're also going to add a fourth set (of 6 reps) for all primary exercises. So, while your biceps and triceps routines go up from 6 to 7 sets each, your chest, back, shoulder, and upper leg routines will each jump from 9 to 14. Finally, we're also adding a third exercise to your abdominal routine.

You're still in charge: You can do 3 sets of any ab exercise you choose, but instead of doing a fixed number of reps, you're going to do your sets of this last ab exercise *to failure*. That means you'll do as many reps as you can until you absolutely can do no more. Believe me, you'll want to choose that third ab exercise carefully.

You've probably realized that with the freedom of choosing your own exercises comes responsibility. While you could pick the exercises that are easiest for you and repeat them every week, you won't be getting much out of the program that way. Muscles only stay strong and toned when they're regularly challenged, so you've got to keep mixing in the exercises that you find more difficult—*and* you've got to attack your muscle groups from all angles, being sure to target every muscle and muscle part regularly.

Over time, your muscles will find the easiest way to perform any movement, so you've got to constantly change your workout if you want to continue to grow and improve. After all, growth and improvement are the real goals of this fitness program. (Come to think of it, those are pretty good goals to have in life, too.)

LEVEL 4 PROGRAM

Exercise Schedule
Number of Sets and Reps, Rest Intervals, and Weight Schemes

PROGRAM DURATION: 28 days

WORKOUT FREQUENCY: 4 days a week

PRIMARY EXERCISES

4 sets of 12, 10, 8, and 6 reps

90-second maximum rest between sets

Increase weight each set

SECONDARY EXERCISES

3 sets of 15, 12, and 10 reps

60-second maximum rest between sets

Increase weight each set

CALF EXERCISES

First Exercise: 4 sets of 12, 10, 8, and 6 reps

Second Exercise: 3 sets of 15, 12,
    and 10 reps

60-second maximum rest between sets

Increase weight each set

ABDOMINAL EXERCISES

First and Second Exercises: 3 sets of
    15–20 reps

Third Exercise: 3 sets to failure

60-second maximum rest between sets

NOTE: Pick your primary and secondary exercises from the master list located on pages 83–85.

DAY 1	DAY 2	DAY 3	DAY 4	DAY 5	DAY 6	DAY 7

BACK
2 primary
2 secondary
 	
ABS
1 upper or
  upper/middle
  abs
1 lower abs
1 your choice
	SHOULDERS
	2 primary
	2 secondary
	
	TRICEPS
	1 primary
	1 secondary
	
	ABS
	1 upper or
	  upper/middle
	  abs
	1 lower abs
	1 your choice
		OFF	UPPER LEGS
			2 primary
			2 secondary
			
			CALVES
			2 exercises
				CHEST
				2 primary
				2 secondary
				
				BICEPS
				1 primary
				1 secondary
				
				ABS
				1 upper or
				  upper/middle
				  abs
				1 lower abs
				1 your choice
					OFF	OFF

Level 4: Sample Week

DAY 1	DAY 2	DAY 3
BACK (14 sets) **Primary** **Bent-Over Row–Barbell** 4 sets of 12, 10, 8, and 6 reps **Row–T-Bar** 4 sets of 12, 10, 8, and 6 reps **Secondary** **Lat Pull-Down–Front** 3 sets of 15, 12, and 10 reps **Good Morning–Barbell** 3 sets of 15, 12, and 10 reps **ABS** (6 sets) **Upper Abs** **Crunch** 3 sets of 15–20 reps **Lower Abs** **Hanging Leg Raise** 3 sets of 15–20 reps **Your Choice** **Reverse Crunch or** **Lying Leg Raise** 3 sets to failure	**SHOULDERS** (14 sets) **Primary** **Front Military Press–** **Barbell** 3 sets of 12, 10, 8, and 6 reps **Shoulder Press–** **Dumbbell** 3 sets of 12, 10, 8, and 6 reps **Secondary** **Front Raise–Dumbbell** 3 sets of 15, 12, and 10 reps **Side Raise–Dumbbell** 3 sets of 15, 12, and 10 reps **TRICEPS** (7 sets) **Primary** **Skullcrushers–Barbell** 3 sets of 12, 10, 8, and 6 reps **Secondary** **Kickback–Dumbbell** 3 sets of 15, 12, and 10 reps **ABDOMINALS** (9 sets) **Upper/Middle Abs** **Seated Crunch–Rope** 3 sets of 15–20 reps **Lower Abs** **Leg Raise–Vertical** **Bench** 3 sets of 15–20 reps **Your Choice** **Hanging Twisting** **Leg Raise** 3 sets to failure	OFF

DAY 4	DAY 5	DAY 6	DAY 7
UPPER LEGS (14 sets) **Primary** **Squat–Barbell** 4 sets of 12, 10, 8, and 6 reps **Leg Press–Machine** 4 sets of 12, 10, 8, and 6 reps **Secondary** **Prone Hamstring Curl–** **Dumbbell** 3 sets of 15, 12, and 10 reps **Standing Hamstring** **Curl–Machine** 3 sets of 15, 12, and 10 reps **CALVES** (7 sets) **Standing Calf Raise–** **Machine** 4 sets of 12, 10, 8, and 6 reps **Seated Calf Raise–** **Machine** 3 sets of 15, 12, and 10 reps	**CHEST** (14 sets) **Primary** **Bench Press–Barbell** 4 sets of 12, 10, 8, and 6 reps **Incline Press–Barbell** 4 sets of 12, 10, 8, and 6 reps **Secondary** **Incline Fly–Dumbbell** 3 sets of 15, 12, and 10 reps **Cable Crossover** 3 sets of 15, 12, and 10 reps **BICEPS** (7 sets) **Primary** **Biceps Curl–Barbell** 4 sets of 12, 10, 8, and 6 reps **Secondary** **Concentration Curl–** **Dumbbell** 3 sets of 15, 12, and 10 reps **ABS** (9 sets) **Upper/Middle Abs** **Kneeling Crunch–Rope** 3 sets of 15–20 reps **Lower Abs** **Leg Raise–Bench** 3 sets of 15–20 reps **Your Choice** **Seated Twist** 3 sets to failure	OFF	OFF

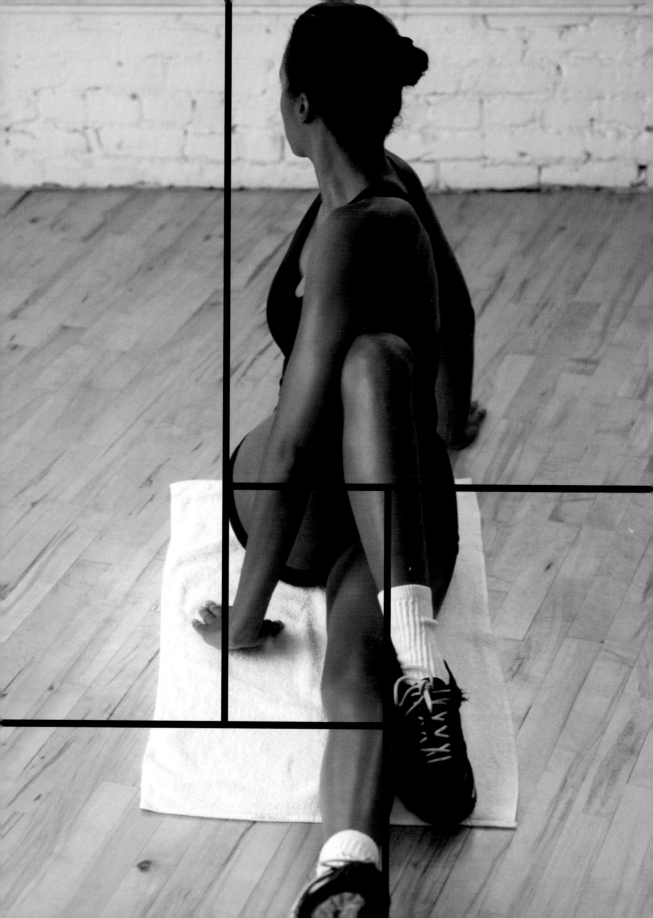

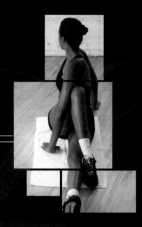

CHAPTER 10

LEVEL 5
(Expert)

This is a chapter for total fitness pros and professional bodybuilders. Please be careful if you're not one of these types because these workouts are *not* for amateurs.

As for the few of you out there at that level, let me just say thanks for buying my book. You're buff, tough, but can't get enough. At this point, you've truly mastered all of the exercises in this book: You're completely familiar with the movements, you know what you need to do to maintain perfect form, and you've even learned advanced tips for how to get the most out of every rep. You clearly know exactly which exercises to use to target virtually every muscle group or part of your body, which has given you tremendous control over the shape of your body and its proportions. You also understand how to schedule your workouts and how to structure them to meet your own individual needs and goals.

You've worked hard and have achieved your physical goals (as well as some mental ones). Be proud! You're a success, and to remain successful, you only need to continue doing what you've been doing in Level 4, with the same intensity.

But if you want more—that is, if you want to continue to build and refine your body, increase your strength, and further exceed your limits, there are a few more things you can learn. In this part of the book, I'll let you in on the special techniques that advanced weight trainers utilize to take their workouts—and their physiques—to the next level. These methods have been designed for and by competitive bodybuilders. Remember, only extremely fit people and body-builders should do these exercises. They're among the toughest you'll find anywhere.

Level 5 describes a wealth of expert weight-training strategies, including my own favorites, to help you shock your body into continued progress. So if you're still with me, let's get to it!

Crazy—and It Works

I'll be the first to tell you that some of the techniques and routines in this chapter may seem completely insane. Some of my fellow trainers will disagree about the effectiveness of some of these techniques, but that's to be expected. Everybody is different, and every *body* is different— different exercises work for different people. The same is certainly true for these expert tech-niques. Through trial and error, you'll find what works best for you.

Over the years, people in gyms have told me that I shouldn't spend so much time doing squats, or that I was lifting too much weight a lot of the time. I politely thanked them for their advice, but I didn't follow it—because only I know what I can do and what I want to achieve.

Think about what you want to achieve. I'll be honest here—some of these workouts have pushed me so far beyond my limits that I've vomited after some incredibly grueling sets; oth-ers left me so sore that walking was painful for a week. But nothing says that *you* have to work that hard. You can decide how far to push yourself with any of these expert techniques. It was my own will and determination to reach my goals that pushed me to those extremes. I'm also certain that if I hadn't incorporated these methods into my workout on occasion, I'd never look the way I do. What I'm trying to say is this: Sometimes it will take an extraordinary workout to get extraordinary results.

Now, let me give you a little advice. These techniques aren't for the weak, and I certainly don't recommend them for people who aren't going to give 100%. Let me also give a warn-ing to all of the overeager overachievers out there: The techniques and routines described in this chapter are *not* to be used for every exercise or every workout. If you follow these routines all of the time, your body will have a tough time recuperating. You'll be over-training and, just as surely as if you weren't using these expert techniques at all, your gains will stop. These routines are to be performed by fitness experts to shake up their workouts, and to shock the body into new development. I repeat: If you use some of the techniques and routines from this chapter in every workout, you'll burn yourself out. Did you ever hear the expression "too much of a good thing"?

Expert Techniques

These advanced methods will allow you to intensify both your workouts and individual exercises for maximum gains. There are five basic ways you can do this:

1. **Manipulate the repetitions in a set.** Increase or decrease the number of reps performed, change the speed at which they're performed, or continue until absolute failure (when you just can't do one more) or beyond failure (with assistance).

2. **Increase or decrease the amount of weight lifted.** This generally changes in inverse proportion to the number of reps attempted: When we increase the number of reps, we use less weight; when we do fewer reps, we lift more.

3. **Increase or decrease the number of sets done.**

4. **Limit or eliminate rest between sets or exercises.**

5. **Change the order of exercises.** Pair or combine exercises to be done consecutively.

Individually, these five methods can significantly boost the intensity of your workouts; by combining them, their effectiveness is multiplied. That's why you'll find that all of the methods discussed in this chapter employ multiple techniques at once. When you simultaneously change a number of variables in an exercise or workout, you're much more likely to shock the muscle or muscle group into renewed growth. Allow me to further explain what I mean.

Partial Reps (Burns)

Partial reps are half- or quarter-movements that you do at the end of a set when you're already at the point of failure or when you simply can't do another full rep. They sometimes look silly, but you need to get over that. Partial reps will take the muscle or muscle group you're training to a whole new level of muscle fatigue—you might call it "super-failure"—and give you a superior pump.

I sometimes use partial reps when I'm working my middle deltoids with the **Side raise–dumbbell** exercise. I choose a weight that I can usually do a set of 12 reps with, and I continue until I can no longer do a full rep. Then, without resting, I try to squeeze out another rep, maintaining good form as I slowly lift the dumbbells up as far as I can. A whole rep isn't going to happen—but I can do a partial rep, and maybe another, smaller one after that. I continue to do smaller and smaller partial reps until I can't lift the dumbbells at all. That's when I know I'm done.

After a set with partial reps, you'll feel a warm sensation in the muscle or muscle group you're working, which is why they're also called "burns." That burning sensation means you've stimulated muscle fibers that you probably haven't been hitting with your standard sets. Good. That's what we're trying to do with all of these expert techniques.

Forced Reps

Forced reps take the partial-rep method to the next level. This technique is very simple, but you can't do it alone. To do forced reps, you'll need your training partner to help you complete an extra rep or two at the end of your set—after the muscle or muscle group you're working has reached the point of fatigue. I'm sure you've seen this technique used in the gym a million times, especially on the bench press. Instead of just watching to make sure that the pressers don't drop the bar on their necks, the spotters actually help them squeeze an extra rep or two out of the set by helping them lift the bar.

Be sure to select a good training partner for forced reps. In the interest of safety, any spotter should be strong enough to handle the weight themselves if necessary, and he or she needs to focus completely on what you're doing for the entire exercise. For forced reps, a *really* good training partner will be careful not to help you lift until you've reached the point of failure, and at that point he or she will lift just enough so that you can barely complete another rep or two.

To get the most out of forced reps, your training partner has to be tuned in to exactly what you can and cannot do.

Forced reps are great for helping you gradually increase the weight you lift from workout to workout. Ideally, it works like this: If this week you can do 6 reps of an exercise by yourself, followed by 2 forced reps; next week you'll be able to do 8 reps of that same weight by yourself, followed by 2 forced reps. The next week, you'll be able to move up in weight and do 6 reps yourself, followed by 2 forced reps, and so on. Forced reps are all about making steady progress.

Pause Reps (Rest Reps)

Picture an exercise. Now picture the weight you usually lift for the last set of that exercise—a weight that will barely let you do 6 reps. Today, you're going to do *10* reps with that weight. How in the world will you be able to do this? The answer is: pause reps.

The scientific theory behind this technique is that a muscle recovers 90% of its strength just 10 seconds after you finish exerting it. So, with pause reps, we're going to rest for 10 seconds between every rep. Pause reps, which are also called "rest reps," will allow you to use heavier weights in your sets.

I sometimes use pause reps to intensify my chest workout. Since I have to be completely warmed up to use this technique, I use it on my last set of bench presses. I'll use a weight that I ordinarily have trouble lifting 6 times—for me, that's 365 pounds. I'll do my first rep with no problems, put the bar back on the rack, and wait 10 seconds. Then I'll do another rep. I try to follow this rep-pause pattern for 10 reps.

Don't be fooled by all that resting; pause reps are intense. I recommend that you have someone spot you with these. (Of course, as you know, whenever you use heavy weights, you should use a spotter.) If I can't get the weight up for the final two reps, I do forced reps with the help of my training partner.

Pause reps are great for getting your body accustomed to heavier weights. They really help get you past plateaus or sticking points, which is when you get stuck doing an exercise at a certain weight for a long time and can't seem to get past it. Pause reps will help you break through that barrier, add weight, and get you to the next level.

Different Rep Schemes

Over the years I've used many different rep schemes in my workouts. I'm a firm believer in the effectiveness of the pyramid-rep pattern we used in Levels 2–4. I use that rep scheme as the base of my entire workout. As you know, in the pyramid system, you start with a lighter weight and a high rep count and add weight every set as you reduce the number of repetitions. For example, you repeat sets of an exercise with 12 reps at 200 pounds, 10 reps at 220 pounds, 8 reps at 240 pounds, and so on. I don't think that there's a better rep pattern to help you build a solid physical foundation than the 12-10-8-6 pyramid.

However, sometimes you need to deviate from the standard pyramid and shake up your rep scheme to shock your body into new growth. I was very fortunate as a teenager to train with some Olympic weight lifters, who taught me a lot of different rep schemes—and let me tell you, each one was harder than the next. Many times, after I've used one of these alternate-rep schemes in my leg workout, I practically have to crawl out to my car.

Here are some examples of popular alternate-rep schemes that you can use to wake up your muscles and avoid plateaus. *Do not use these rep schemes for every workout.* Stick with the pyramid system as the base of your regular workouts, then try one of these schemes every so often to expand your limits:

1. 10 Sets of 20

I've often used this rep pattern for squats. I use the same weight for the entire 10 sets and stick to the standard 60-second rest between sets. By the time I finish the 10th set, I don't know whether to fall down, cry, or throw up. This rep scheme is extremely brutal—besides muscular strength, you need to have incredible stamina. You can use this rep scheme for any exercise, but I recommend using it for your most basic and complex primary exercises, such as squats, bench presses, and bent-over rows.

2. 10 Sets of 10

This is a great method for increasing your focus. Drop your regular workout schedule for a day and use this rep scheme for a full-body workout. Pick just one exercise for each body part—I recommend that you use primary exercises here—and do 10 sets of 10 reps for every exercise. Again, you should use the same weight throughout the entire 10 sets.

I use the "10 sets of 10" system a lot. Sometimes, instead of using it for a full-body workout, I'll apply the rep scheme to some of the exercises in my regular workout that day. For example, if I'm training my chest, I'll do 10 sets of 10 for the bench press, then use the standard pyramid system for my incline press and flys. How you use this rep scheme is up to you, since you're the only one who knows how much your body can handle. I guarantee you'll spice up any workout if you use this scheme for one exercise. Just be sure to pick a weight that's heavy enough to be challenging—don't baby yourself.

3. 6 Sets of 6

This low-rep, heavyweight plan is a good rep scheme for increasing your strength on primary exercises. Early in my weight-training career, I was on a quest to reach a 1-rep max of 500 pounds on the bench press. Growing up in Long Island, a place that seems to be overrun with bodybuilders, there was always competition at the gym, and it usually involved the bench press. Using this unusual scheme, I was able to leave many of my bench-pressing peers in the dust.

I'd use a weight to the point that I could just barely do 6 sets of 6 reps. Then, during my next chest workout, I'd increase the weight by 5 pounds and try to repeat the pattern. When I could do this—and most weeks I was able to—I knew that I could try 5 more pounds the next time.

If I got stuck at a certain weight and couldn't do 6 sets of 6, I'd stay with that weight, week in and week out, until I could. I used this scheme for 3 months and added 30 pounds to my bench press—I wasn't achieving those results with the standard pyramid system.

4. High Reps

Weight training at the expert level is largely geared toward lifting ever-increasing amounts of weight week after week. It follows that switching to a high-rep scheme is often a great way to stimulate your muscles. I've often used high-rep sets myself: I've done sets of 40, 50, or 100 reps—you name it.

When I diet down for a photo shoot, I stay away from the heavy weights I usually lift. Instead, I choose high-rep sets to shock my muscles. I usually do 1 high-rep set for each muscle group. For example, on biceps day, I might add a high-rep set to the end of my regular **Biceps curl–barbell** routine. I'll do 4 sets of 12, 10, 8, and 6 reps, and then I'll finish my biceps off with a set of 30–40 reps. I often can't lift my arms after that set. I've also used high-rep sets on the **Leg extension–machine** for quads, the **Cable crossover** for chest, and the **Squat–machine** for legs. High-rep sets have also been very useful in getting my stubborn calves to grow. You can also use a high-rep scheme for an entire body workout—it's up to you how and when you want to work these sets into your workouts.

Here's my favorite high-rep workout:

UPPER LEGS

Leg Press–Machine (Primary)

1 set of 15 reps at 945 lbs., followed by a 60-second rest

1 set of 20 reps at 765 lbs., followed by a 60-second rest

1 set of 20 reps at 585 lbs., followed by a 60-second rest

2 set of 40 reps at 405 lbs., followed by a 60-second rest

(I was using this routine when I weighed about 275 pounds. I use the same system now, but with considerably lighter weights.)

5. Low Reps

Low-rep schemes are a great way to increase your strength in certain lifts. Power-lifters, including Olympic weight lifters, use sets of extremely low reps to help them build their strength. Doing low-rep sets makes perfect sense for them since their primary goal is to increase their 1-rep max—after all, they only have to lift a weight once in their lifetime to set a world record or win a gold medal.

I don't recommend low-rep schemes to everybody because lifting the heavy weights involved pushes your body to its limits on almost every set, significantly increasing your risk of injury. If you do 1-rep sets, don't do them frequently, and make sure that you have a strong and attentive spotter when you do. Even college and professional football players generally keep their rep schemes between 10 and 14 reps. This is because team trainers want their athletes in shape—not hurt. If you have a multimillion-dollar player pushing out one rep for every exercise, eventually he's going to injure himself.

Here's a low-rep scheme I've used:

BACK
Dead-Lift–Barbell (Primary)

1 set of 6 reps at 455 lbs., followed by a 60-second rest

1 set of 4 reps at 500 lbs., followed by a 60-seond rest

1 set of 3 reps at 525 lbs., followed by a 60-second rest

1 set of 1–2 reps at 550 lbs., followed by a 60-second rest

1 set of 1 rep at 560 lbs., followed by a 60-second rest.

6. 21s

This unique rep scheme combines partial reps and full reps into a very challenging tri-set. Twenty-ones are excellent for stimulating all of the different areas of a single muscle, such as biceps, triceps, quadriceps, hamstrings, or any of the 3 heads of the deltoids. In a 21, you perform 7 half-reps of the first half of an exercise motion, then another 7 half-reps of the second half of the motion, and finish with 7 full reps of the exercise. The 3 groups of 7 reps are performed without any rest in between them.

The only time I do 21s is when I want to shock my biceps. It's a great way to intensify the **Biceps curl–barbell** exercise. I start off by curling the weight from the bottom to midpoint for 7 reps. With no rest, I continue to curl, but this time I curl the weight from midpoint of the motion to the top. Then, with no rest, I finish off the set by doing 7 complete reps.

This technique provides a killer workout. Your biceps will feel as if they're ready to pop after a set of 21s. You can do 6 half-reps of an exercise, followed immediately by another 6 half-reps and 6 full reps and call them 18s—you can even do 27s or 33s if you want to. But I wouldn't recommend doing more than 2 sets of any of these—if you do, you'll burn yourself out. Anyway, if you do them right, you won't be able to do more than 2 sets.

Pre-Exhaustion

Pre-exhaustion is when you reverse the usual order of your workout and perform an exercise that tightly targets one muscle in a muscle group—or one part of a single muscle—before you perform a more complex exercise. It usually involves doing a secondary exercise before a primary, or a secondary before a more complex secondary. The point of pre-exhaustion is to fatigue a muscle part right before you work the entire muscle, or an individual muscle right before you work the entire muscle group it's in. The change in order makes both of the exercises more effective, as you'll be able to do more reps or more weight than usual on the first exercise, and the second exercise will be more difficult than usual because the muscle or muscle group isn't fresh. Both effects will shock your muscles into new growth.

Here are some examples of pre-exhaustion combinations I use:

UPPER LEGS

Leg Extension–Machine (Secondary)

3 sets of 20 reps, with a 60-second rest after each

Squat–Barbell (Primary)

4 sets of 10, 8, 6, and 4 reps, with a 60-second rest after each

SHOULDERS

Side Raise–Dumbbell (Secondary)

3 sets of 12, 10, and 8 reps, with a 60-second rest after each

Front Military Press–Barbell (Primary)

3 sets of 10, 8, and 6 reps, with a 60-second rest after each

ABDOMINALS

Crunch (Upper Abs)

3 sets of 20 reps, with a 60-second rest after each

Leg Raise–Bench (Lower Abs)

3 sets to failure, with a 60-second rest after each

Super Sets

While this absolutely essential technique is likely to turn you into a Man or Woman of Steel, the name has nothing to do with Superman. Super-setting happens when you perform sets of 2 different exercises consecutively without resting. You can do super sets focusing on a single muscle group or pairing exercises for different muscle groups—it's commonly done both ways. If you combine exercises for different muscle groups, you'll get the most bang for your buck. It also helps to pair exercises for opposing muscles or muscle groups: quadriceps and hamstrings, chest and back, biceps and triceps.

Here are examples of a couple of my favorite super-set routines:

SINGLE MUSCLE GROUP–BICEPS
Biceps Curl–Barbell (Primary)
1 set of 10 reps, followed immediately by:
Concentration Curl–Dumbbell (Secondary)
1 set of 10 reps
Preacher Curl–Barbell (Secondary)
1 set of 20 reps, followed immediately by:
Standing Hammer Curl–Dumbbell (Secondary)
1 set of 20 reps
Biceps Curl–Dumbbell (Primary)
1 set of 6 reps, followed immediately by:
Preacher Curl–Barbell (Secondary)
1 set of 12 reps

OPPOSING MUSCLE GROUPS–CHEST/BACK
Bench Press–Barbell (Primary)
1 set of 10 reps, followed immediately by:
Chin-Up (Primary)
1 set to failure
Incline Press–Barbell (Primary)
1 set of 20 reps, followed immediately by:
One-Arm Row–Dumbbell (Primary)
1 set of 10 reps
Bench Press–Dumbbell (Primary)
1 set of 6 reps, followed immediately by:
Lat Pull-Down–Front (Secondary)
1 set of 20 reps

Tri-Sets

I'm sure you know that the prefix *tri* means "three." Tri-sets kick it up a notch beyond super sets because in a tri-set, you choose 3 exercises for the same muscle group and do sets of each consecutively with no rest in between. Tri-sets are great for people with limited time because they provide a very short and intense workout. I often rely on them when I'm traveling and have limited time to spend in the gym.

Here's an example of one of my tri-set routines:

TRICEPS
Narrow-Grip Bench Press–Barbell (Primary)
1 set of 12 reps, followed immediately by:
Two-Arm Cable Push-Down–Straight Bar (Primary)
1 set of 10 reps, followed immediately by:
Skullcrushers–Barbell (Primary)
1 set to failure

Giant Sets

This technique is definitely not for the faint of heart. Forget doing 3 exercises in a row—in a giant set, you'll do 4. (So why aren't they called "quad sets"? Probably because your quadriceps are often referred to as "quads" for short.) You'll choose 4 exercises for the same muscle group and do 6 of each consecutively with no rest in between. Can you say "taxing"? During my competitive bodybuilding days, I used to do 3 giant sets for my upper legs—that's a total of 12 sets with only 2 rest periods among them—and I used to see stars after I was done. If you do giant sets, give them 100% of your effort, but listen carefully to your body to avoid injury.

Here's one of my giant-set routines:

QUADRICEPS
Squat–Barbell (Primary)
1 set of 10 reps, followed immediately by:
Leg Press–Machine (Primary)
1 set of 10 reps, followed immediately by:
Hack Squat–Machine (Primary)
1 set of 10 reps, followed immediately by:
Leg Extension–Machine (Secondary)
1 set of 20 or more

Strip Sets/Drop Sets/Down-the-Rack Sets

No, these sets don't involve a stripper's pole, but they *are* better when you do them with a friend. In a strip set, you'll do multiple sets of one exercise without resting. After you've performed each set to failure, you or your spotter will quickly remove a plate or two from the bar or machine to reduce the weight. You'll then immediately proceed right on to the next set. Strip sets allow you to take the muscle you're training beyond the point of normal failure. To follow this technique when you're using a heavy bar or plate-loaded machine, you really need a spotter to keep the intervals between sets to a minimum.

If you're training alone, it's easier and faster to do strip sets on a machine with a weight stack. To reduce the weight between sets, all you have to do is move the pin up the stack. When training alone, it's also easier to follow this technique with dumbbell exercises. When you're using dumbbells, they're called "down-the-rack sets" because you move down the rack as you switch dumbbells to reduce weight. Call them whatever you want—strip sets, drop sets, or down-the-rack sets—they all work the same way. Do a set to failure, reduce the weight, do another set to failure, reduce the weight, and so on. It's up to you to figure out how many sets you can handle.

Here are examples of my strip-set, drop-set, and down-the-rack set routines:

STRIP SET—CHEST

Bench Press—Barbell (Primary)

1 set at 365 lbs. to failure (about 6 reps), followed by no rest

1 set at 335 lbs. to failure, followed by no rest

1 set at 305 lbs. to failure, followed by no rest

1 set at 225 lbs. to failure; rest.

DROP SET—UPPER LEGS (HAMSTRINGS)
Leg Extension—Machine (Secondary)

1 set at a weight of your choice to failure (about 12 reps), followed by no rest

1 set at a weight of your choice to failure, followed by no rest

1 set at 40 lbs. to failure, followed by no rest

1 set at 60 lbs. to failure, followed by no rest

1 set at 80 lbs. to failure; rest

This is a great burn for your legs.

DOWN-THE-RACK SET—BICEPS

Biceps Curl–Barbell (Secondary)

1 set at 70 lbs. to failure, followed by no rest

1 set at 60 lbs to failure, followed by no rest

1 set at 50 lbs to failure, followed by no rest

1 set at 40 lbs to failure, followed by no rest

1 set at 30 lbs. to failure; rest

After this, my biceps are so exhausted that I can barely lift my arms.

Staggered Sets

This is a great way to bring weak or underdeveloped muscle groups up to par with the rest of your fantastic physique. Staggered sets add a cardio component to your weight training, yet don't add a single minute to your gym time! They're sets of unrelated exercises that you do between sets of the exercises in your regular workout. For example, let's say that you have weak calf muscles—staggered sets are a great way to get in some extra work and turn those "calves" into "beef." Instead of resting between sets of bench presses on chest day or biceps curls on biceps day, you'll squeeze in some extra calf exercises, which won't take anything away from your chest or biceps workouts. Those muscles will still get their rest between sets, and your calves will get the extra work they need.

Staggered sets work best if you use them to help develop small muscle groups or individual muscles: calves, biceps, triceps, hamstrings, quadriceps, rear deltoids, middle deltoids, or front deltoids. Here's an example:

CALF STAGGERED SETS ON CHEST DAY

Bench Press–Barbell (Primary)

Seated Calf Raise–Machine

Sets of each exercise alternated without rest

Incline Press–Barbell (Primary)

Standing Calf Raise–Machine

Sets of each exercise alternated without rest

Instinctive Training

Of all the techniques listed in this chapter, this is the most difficult to master and can't even be taught. Basically, instinctive training means that your regular workout schedule goes out the window. Instead, you train as often as you want, exercising whichever body part or parts you like, and working them as hard as you want. You base your training on how you feel and what you think your body needs. For example, if it's leg day and your legs are sore, you'll listen to your body and train something else.

Instinctive training is only for the most advanced and devoted weight trainers. To really make this technique work for you, you have to know your body inside and out, and you have to have a strong work ethic. Otherwise, it's much too easy to simply be lazy about your fitness regimen and call it "instinctive training."

My favorite expert workouts are as follows:

Expert Chest Workout

PARTIAL REPS (BURNS)
Bench Press–Barbell (Primary)

3 regular sets of 12, 10, and 8 reps—each set followed by a 60-second rest, then 1 set of 6 reps followed by no rest, and 1 set of 20 partial reps.

SUPER SETS
Incline Press–Dumbbell (Primary)
Incline Fly–Dumbbell (Secondary)

4 super sets of 6–15 reps of each exercise—no rest between the 2 exercises, and a 60-second rest after each exercise pair.

SUPER SETS WITH HIGH REPS
Cable Crossover (Secondary)
Dip–Parallel Bars (Primary)

3 super sets of 25–30 reps of the **Crossover**, followed immediately by the **Dip** to failure—with a 60-second rest after each exercise pair.

Expert Back Workout

STANDARD SETS

Chin-Up (Primary)

3 sets to failure, with a 60-second rest after each set.

6 SETS OF 6

Bent-Over Row–Barbell (Primary)

6 sets of 6 reps, with a 60-second rest after each set

SUPER SETS

Front Lat Pull-Down (Secondary)

Rear Lat Pull-Down (Secondary)

3 super sets of 12–15 reps of the **Front lat pull-down;** followed immediately by the **Rear lat pull-down** to failure, with a 60-second rest after each exercise pair.

SUPER SETS

Dead Lift–Barbell (Primary)

Hyperextension–Machine (Secondary)

3 super sets of 8, 6, and 4 reps of the **Dead lift;** followed immediately by the **Hyperextension** to failure, with a 60-second rest after each exercise pair.

SUPER SETS

Shrug–Barbell (Secondary)

Shrug–Dumbbell (Secondary)

3 super sets of 12 or fewer reps of each exercise, with no rest between the 2 exercises, and a 60-second rest after each exercise pair.

Expert Shoulder Workout

STANDARD SETS
Front Military Press–Barbell (Primary)

5 sets of 12, 10, 8, 6, and 4 reps, with a 60-second rest after each set.

PARTIAL REPS (BURNS)
Side Raise–Dumbbell (Secondary)

3 sets of 12, 10, and 8 reps, each set followed immediately by partial reps to failure, with a 60-second rest after each set.

SUPER SETS
Upright Row–Barbell (Primary)

Front Raise–Barbell (Secondary)

3 super sets of 10–15 reps of each exercise, with no rest between the 2 exercises, and a 60-second rest after each exercise pair.

TRI-SETS WITH HIGH REPS
Reverse Fly–Pec Deck (Secondary)

Standing Bent-Over Raise–Dumbbell (Secondary)

Seated Bent-Over Raise–Dumbbell (Secondary)

3 tri-sets of 20–30 reps of each exercise, with no rest between the 3 exercises, and a 60-second rest after each exercise trio.

Expert Arm Workout

I often combine my biceps and triceps workouts into one workout. Since they're opposite muscle groups, combining the workouts provides extra benefits. I usually work first biceps then triceps—you may wish to reverse the order or mix up your exercises to work both muscle groups at the same time. Super sets, which combine biceps and triceps exercises, yield fantastic results for some people.

BICEPS

21s

Biceps Curl–Barbell (Primary)

Two 21-rep sets—7 reps of the bottom half of the curl, followed immediately by 7 reps of the bottom half of the curl, followed immediately by 7 reps of the full curl, with a 60-second rest after each set.

HIGH REPS

Preacher Curl–Barbell (Secondary)

4 sets of 12, 10, 8, and 20 reps, with a 60-second rest after each set.

SUPER SETS

Concentration Curl–Dumbbell (Secondary)
Seated Hammer Curl (Secondary)

3 super sets of 10–15 reps of each exercise, with no rest between the 2 exercises, and a 60-second rest after each exercise pair.

HIGH REPS

Standing Two-Hand Overhead Cable Curl (Secondary)

3 sets of 30 reps, with a 60-second rest after each set.

TRICEPS

GIANT SETS

Two-Arm Cable Push-Down–Straight Bar (Primary)
Narrow-Grip Bench Press–Barbell (Primary)
Kickback–Dumbbell (Secondary)
Triceps Dip–Machine (Primary)

4 giant sets of 15, 12, 10, and 8 reps of each exercise (or to failure), with no rest between the 4 exercises, and a 60-second rest after each giant set.

Expert Total-Leg Workout

Your calves are worked hard whenever you exercise your upper legs, yet I often add a few calf exercises to the end of an upper-leg workout to do a total-leg workout. The pre-exhaustion of your calves on these days will make the calf exercises extra effective.

TRI-SETS WITH HIGH REPS
Squat–Barbell (Primary)
Leg Press–Machine (Primary)
Hack Squat–Machine (Primary)
4 tri-sets of 20, 15, 12, and 10 reps of each exercise (or to failure), with no rest between the 3 exercises, and a 60-second rest after each exercise trio.

STANDARD SETS FOLLOWED BY DROP SETS
Leg Extension–Machine (Secondary)
3 sets of 20, 15, and 12 reps, with a 60-second rest after each set,
then 3 drop sets to failure, with a 60-second rest after each set.

SUPER SETS
Stiff-Legged Dead Lift–Barbell (Secondary)
Standing Hamstring Curl–Machine (Secondary)
3 super-sets to failure on each exercise (10–12 reps each), with no rest between the 2 exercises, and a 60-second rest after each exercise pair.

STANDARD SETS FOLLOWED BY DROP SETS
Prone Hamstring Curl–Dumbbell (Secondary)
4 sets of 15, 12, 10, and 8 reps, with a 60-second rest after each set;
then 4 drop sets to failure, with a 60-second rest after each set.

SUPER SETS
Stiff-Legged Dead Lift–Barbell (Secondary)
Standing Hamstring Curl–Machine (Secondary)
3 super sets to failure on each exercise (10–20 reps each), with no rest between the two exercises, and a 60-second rest after each exercise pair.

SUPER SETS WITH HIGH REPS
Standing Calf Raise–Machine
Seated Calf Raise–Machine
3 super-sets of 25–50 reps of each exercise, with no rest between the 2 exercises, and a 60-second rest after each exercise pair.

Expert Calf Workout

STANDARD SETS
Standing Calf Raise–Machine

3 sets of 6 reps (using heavy weight, obviously), with a 60-second rest after each set.

HIGH REPS
Seated Calf Raise–Machine

3 sets of 30 reps, with a 60-second rest after each set.

SUPER SETS
Donkey Calf Raise–Machine

Toe Raise–Leg Press Machine

4 super-sets to failure on each exercise (10–20 reps each), with no rest between the 2 exercises, and a 60-second rest after each exercise pair.

Expert Abdominal Workout

GIANT SETS
Crunch (Upper Abs)

Leg Raise–Bench (Lower Abs)

Kneeling Crunch–Rope (Upper and Lower Abs)

Hanging Leg Raise (Lower Abs)

4 giant sets to failure on each exercise (10–50 reps each), with no rest between the 4 exercises, and a 60-second rest after each giant set.

HAVE YOU WORKED UP an appetite yet? I know I have! It's time for the food part of the book, so join me in Part IV—Nutrition and The TRUTH.

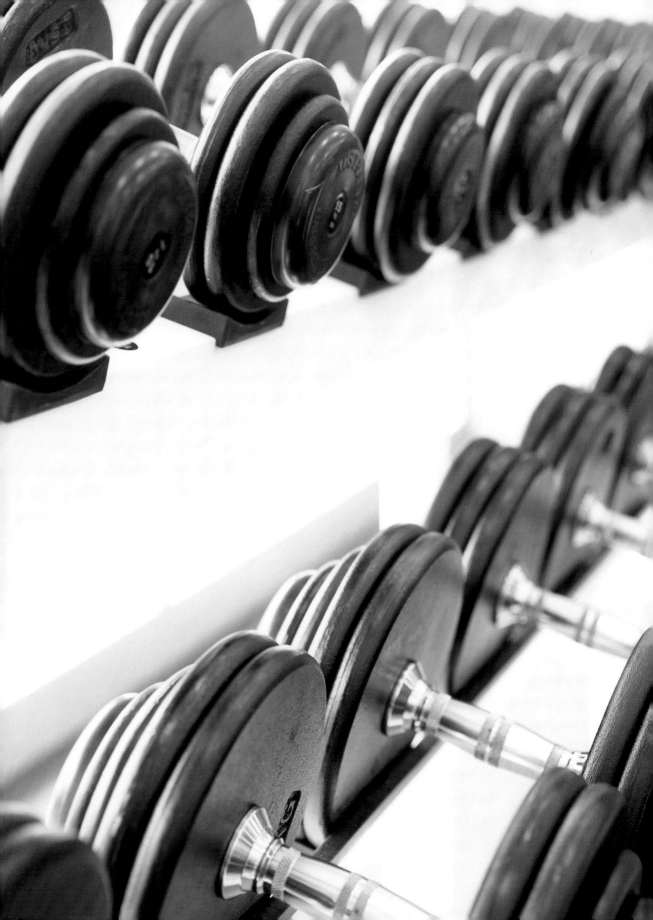

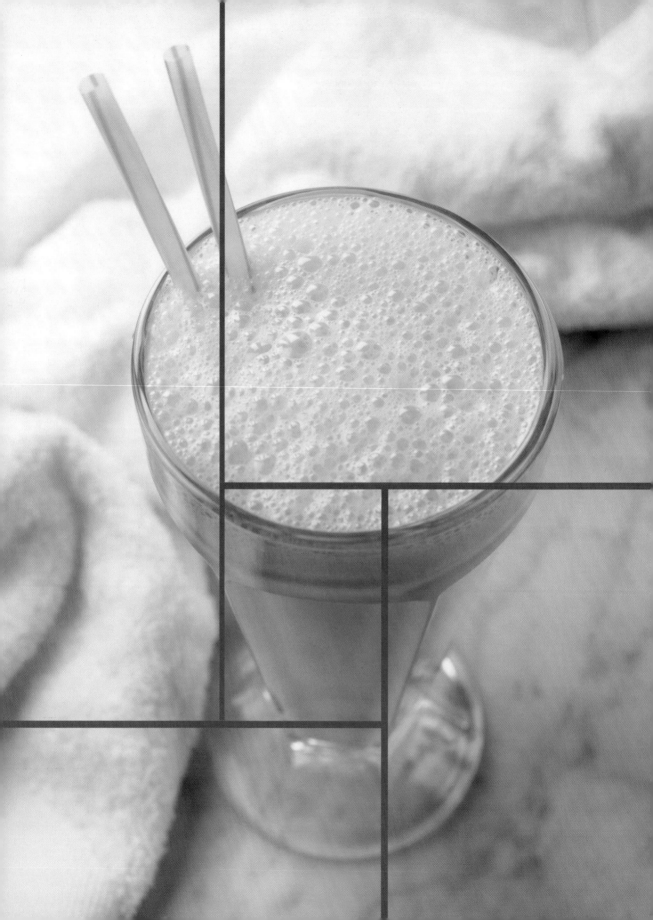

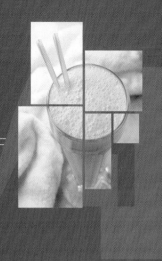

PART III

Nutrition and The TRUTH

Even if you've been working out like a demon, keep in mind that you'll never achieve great results on the outside unless you watch what's on the inside. So it's time to tackle the topic of nutrition, followed by a quick primer of what I do to stay in shape. Finally, if you're sick of listening to me yak, I'll throw in the voices of a few of my clients who will tell you their own remarkable stories about following The TRUTH.

But before we do anything, let's chew on some facts about food.

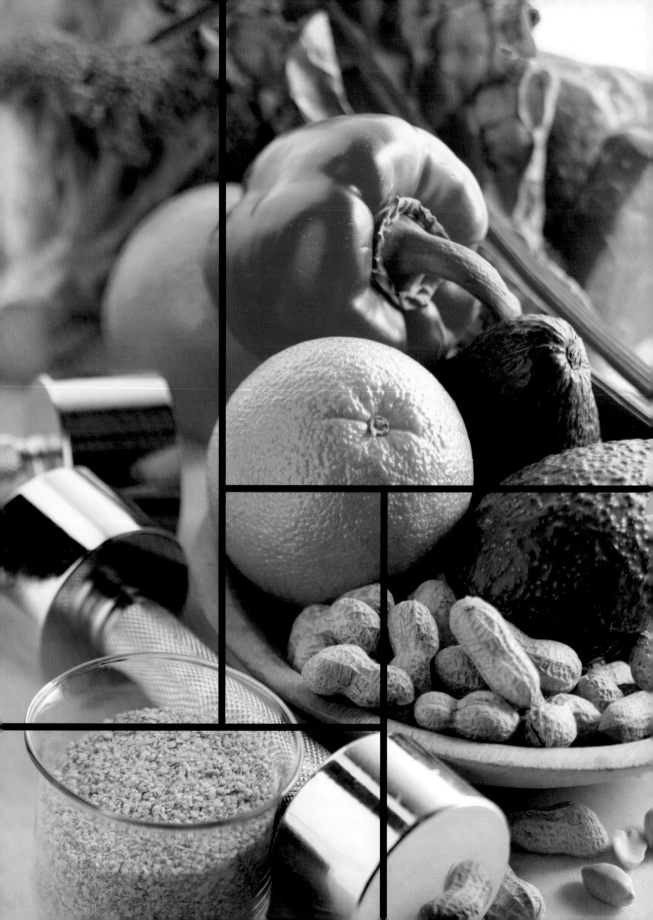

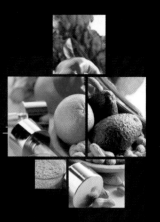

NUTRITION

If you're confused about nutrition and diet, please pull up a bag of yucca chips and pour some cactus juice—or whatever the latest food fad is these days—and pay attention to this section of *The TRUTH*. I know that it seems as if every day somebody discovers a new diet plan to fix our fat problem in a jiffy. The TRUTH program's approach to healthy nutrition is different: It's a clear, simple, realistic, easy, and healthy guide to eating and weight loss. What I propose will also turbo-charge your metabolism as you make "clean eating" a part of your new lifestyle plan.

My plan will work for both men and women because it's based on solid principles of good nutrition. It's an individual plan that you create for yourself with various levels—just like we did in the other parts of this book.

If your idea of a healthy menu includes two all-beef patties, special sauce, lettuce, and cheese, then I suggest that you start at Level 1. However, if you've already incorporated a sound eating program into your life, you can jump to one of the higher levels. No matter where you fall on the healthy-eating spectrum, I've got the tools that will help you look and feel amazing.

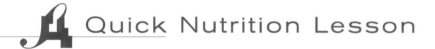 Quick Nutrition Lesson

Wouldn't it be a perfect world if the reward for all of your working out could be a hot-fudge banana split with extra whipped cream on the side? Believe me, I'm just like you—I'd love to bow at the altar of Dairy Queen. Unfortunately, in order to get lean and mean, we have to eat like champs, too.

Here are few things to remember. . . .

Yes, calories count. I'm amazed at the programs out there that tell you to eat limitless amounts of certain types of foods with no regard to caloric intake. There's a simple equation when it comes to weight loss that can't be ignored: If the number of calories you take in exceeds the number of calories you burn, you won't lose weight—you'll gain it. Period.

The reason is simple: A pound of fat equals 3,500 calories. So if you want to lose a pound of fat, you'll have to take in 3,500 fewer calories, burn 3,500 more calories, or adopt some combination of the two over the same period of time.

As you go through this chapter, I'll teach you a very easy way to make sure that you consume the right amount of calories without having to carry around calorie-counting books and a calculator.

Learn the truth about protein, carbohydrates, and fat. Throughout the rest of this book, I'll be referring to these three categories of food nutrients, so it's crucial to understand what their respective functions are. It's also important to make sure that you know how specific foods fit into each category.

Here's a common example: Many people start eating more nuts when trying to raise their protein intake. While nuts do contain protein, the majority of their calories come from fat.

Therefore, I put nuts in the "fat" category, *not* in "protein." To take the guesswork out of all this, and to help you easily understand which foods are in which categories, you'll see a list of protein, carbohydrates, and fat sources in the following chapter.

The key is protein. I believe that protein is the most important nutrient of all. I can almost guarantee that you didn't eat enough protein today—in fact, I'd be willing to bet the house that you haven't eaten enough for about 90% of the days you've been alive. After all, it's easier for most of us to reach for that sugary carbohydrate than a chicken breast.

Why is protein so important? Because it's the only nutrient that actually feeds the lean muscle tissue in your body. If you don't take in enough protein, you'll lose lean muscle tissue. Remember that your goal is to lose body fat, not muscle tissue—without it, your body will lack that toned, shaped appearance that enhances everyone's appearance.

Have you ever seen someone who's lost a lot of weight but doesn't look all that great? They tend to look like a smaller, almost flabbier version of their former self. (I could mention a few top actors, but why get myself in trouble?) These people have lost significant muscle tissue along with their fat, so their skin almost hangs off them because the muscle is no longer there to form the shape of their bodies. This won't happen to you when you follow The TRUTH program because you'll eat adequate protein *and* train properly to maintain and enhance the muscle tissue you currently have. Some examples of high- quality, protein-rich foods include chicken, turkey, fish, egg whites, protein powders, and lean red meat.

Carbs aren't the enemy, but you do have to watch them. As your body's preferred source of energy, the function of carbohydrates is to fuel the body. This is why many people who go on severe low-carb diets often become very lethargic. On the other hand, we've also been told that as long as we're on a very low-fat diet, then we can eat high amounts of carbs and still lose weight.

If you look at the national statistics on rates of obesity, it becomes apparent that as the high-carb philosophy became prevalent, we got fatter as a nation. Why? It's simple: Too many carbs means too many calories, and you know what happens when you eat too many calories—you get fat.

The other problem that many of us experience when eating a lot of carbs is frequent hunger. Those sugary foods tend to be burned by the body very quickly and leave us feeling hungry within an hour or so after we eat them. As you can imagine, we then tend to give in to the hunger by eating more carbs, thus creating a vicious cycle that guarantees weight gain.

We see the opposite extreme with the newly popular low- (or no-) carb diets that allow high amounts of fat and protein. Again, something isn't working because obesity rates are still rising. One of the main problems I have with these diets is the fatigue and lack of energy that many people report. Well, naturally when you deprive the body of its preferred source of energy, you're going to have—you guessed it—less energy! And you can't just shovel as many protein and fat calories as you want into your mouth and hope to lose weight because, once again, you'll be eating way too many calories.

Another concern is that it's almost impossible for most of us to sustain a very low-carbohydrate intake as a long-term lifestyle change. I mean, do you want to go the rest of your life without a bagel? Pasta? Rice? I love good carbs, including fruits, vegetables, whole grains, rice, pasta, breads, and yams. I know that if I were on one of these diets, I'd be searching for something that had a crusty top in my sleep. Then I'd wake up with Wonder Bread wrappers by my feet. It's just not a good way to live.

Fat isn't where it's at—but you do need some of it in your diet. Even though 1 gram of fat contains 9 calories, fats act as a cushion for vital organs, while providing insulation against hot and cold temperatures. Fat also helps maintain and improve the condition of hair, skin, and nails. But most important, fat is another energy source for the body.

Fat also burns slower in your body, which means that you're less likely to be hungry soon after you eat them. Does that mean you should eat lots of fat? No. However, limiting it too much may make losing weight more challenging and require you to fight hunger all the time. I promise that you'll be eating enough fat to provide positive energy and offset hunger, but not so much that you'll gain weight. Plus, just knowing that you get to eat fat should bring a smile to your face!

*L*evel 1: Making the Transition to Healthy Eating in 30 Days

If you haven't been eating healthy (come on . . . don't lie to the guy proposing The TRUTH), this is the place to start. You have to walk before you can run, so consider the next 30 days a nice, easy stroll around the block. By taking these first gradual steps toward healthy eating, you won't lose your mind or shock your body with a drastic program that will be impossible to incorporate into your life.

The next 30 days will prepare you for a lifestyle of healthy eating that will put you in touch with your goals. Just follow my guidelines.

Guideline 1: Healthy Substitutions

All I want you to do at this level is one thing: Stop eating foods that you know aren't healthy and start replacing them with foods that I like to call "clean." Use your common sense to eliminate foods that we all know can't possibly be part of a sound nutritional program. Let me break it down for you: Fried chicken is bad, baked chicken is good. Ben and Jerry aren't your friends—instead, try nonfat frozen yogurt made by some guys with no recognizable names.

To make this easy for you, simply look at the protein, carbohydrate, and fat list provided below. This is the time to trade your poor food choices for healthier ones. For example, don't eat that sausage, but substitute it for healthier protein sources like chicken or turkey.

Let's take a look at a sample day of eating, and how you can make some healthy choices. You won't even believe how many calories you'll save. During this level, you'll just be making little adjustments, which will prime you for bigger changes to come.

Poor Choices

BREAKFAST	Calories
3 eggs	225
Hash browns	320
Buttered bagel	400
Coffee with cream and sugar	100
LUNCH	
Ham and cheese sandwich on white bread with mayo	460
Candy bar	250
Regular cola	200
DINNER	
Chicken caesar salad	630
Dinner roll	214
Chocolate-chip cookie	190
Regular cola	200
SNACK	
1 cup ice cream	500

Total: 3689

Good Choices

BREAKFAST	Calories
5 egg whites	85
Oatmeal	150
Banana	105
Coffee with nonfat creamer and sugar substitute	23
LUNCH	
Turkey sandwich on rye bread with nonfat mayo	328
Apple	81
Sugar-free beverage	0
DINNER	
Grilled chicken breast	215
Yam	160
Large bowl of strawberries	92
Sugar-free beverage	0
SNACK	
1 cup strawberries	46

Total: 1285

Guideline 2: Meal Frequency

Eat 3 meals per day. Feel free to add a snack when you get hungry, but be sure to pick smart snacks such as fresh fruit.

Guideline 3: Cheat Meals

One day a week, you're entitled to have one meal of anything that you want to eat. *Anything.* Pizza? Yes. Cheeseburger and French fries? You got it. Ice cream for dessert? Indulge! Whatever you want is yours, once a week. Just don't do it more than once every 7-day period and you'll be fine. Yes, I'm serious.

The cheat meal serves many positive purposes. First, let's talk about the psychological reality of eating for weight loss. When you start most programs, you're told to eat a certain way until you reach your goals. Sure it sounds good, but when you take a closer look, you come to realize that if you need to lose 50 pounds of fat, you aren't going to get to eat anything you crave for at least the next *6 months*.

Let's get real—even *I* don't have that kind of willpower. In fact, I've never met anyone with that kind of discipline. No matter what people try to tell you, I can virtually guarantee that you'll go off your program more than once a week unless you get some kind of leeway. So a cheat meal every week will actually have the effect of limiting how often you deviate. Now, instead of being loaded with guilt after you stray, you'll simply feel that you enjoyed a meal you earned by staying true to your program.

Think about it: *You'll never be deprived of what you're craving for more than 6 days.* That's not half bad! And, as you progress to the next 2 levels of healthy eating, you'll see that the number of cheat meals will actually increase, not decrease.

Now let's talk about the physical/metabolic benefit of the cheat meal. Your body is incredibly adaptive, with an amazing ability to get used to different stimuli and physical changes. The problem is that when you change your eating patterns to create weight loss, your body gets used to the new program after a short time and starts to accept your new way of eating as a maintenance program instead of a weight-reduction program. This translates into your getting results for a while and then watching the weight loss slow to a grinding halt as your body adjusts to the new program. Your metabolism can actually slow down as this process occurs, and you'll become terribly frustrated.

Believe it or not, your cheat meal can help offset this metabolic nightmare. When you have a high-calorie meal of foods that your body hasn't had on a regular basis, this can have the effect of shocking your metabolism back into action. Your calories for that day will end up higher than normal, which also shocks your metabolism. When you return to your diet the next day, you'll experience a caloric deficiency from the prior day's eating. Your body should respond by dropping some more weight.

Finally, the cheat meal will allow you to keep some sort of normalcy in your life. Want to have a social outing with your friends, significant other, or family every week? Go right ahead—just make it the same day that you take your cheat meal. Do you have a hot date next weekend, and you'd rather not watch what you eat while you're gazing into his or her eyes? No problem. Enjoy your cheat meal that night. As you can see, the cheat meal allows you to follow The TRUTH as a long-term lifestyle, not just as a short-term quick fix.

Level 2: Getting Serious

Now that you've cleaned the poor food choices out of your eating plan and have learned how to make better choices, we can begin to put some structure and more rewards into your meal planning. You're ready to start Level 2 eating and get serious—and that means more results!

What follows is my step-by-step approach for success.

Step 1: Determine Your Personal Daily Nutrient Requirements

The first step in creating your personalized eating plan is to determine the appropriate daily amount of each of the major nutrients we discussed above. The first thing you'll need to know is exactly what you weigh. Once you have that number, simply plug it into the following formulas:

1 gram of protein per body weight

1 gram of carbohydrates per body weight

.22 grams of fat x body weight

These numbers were created by first making a determination of how much protein a person who's training on a regular basis needs to consume in order to properly feed their muscle tissue. When you're working out with weights, you're actually breaking down muscle tissue. As the muscle recuperates and repairs, it comes back stronger and better developed. However, you need protein to help with the process—in fact, it's vital to your success. As you go up in levels in your training, you'll add more protein to your diet. It also helps satisfy your appetite with nutrients that are less calorie-dense than fats and less prone to insulin release and overeating (blame carbs for those two whammies). Speaking of carbs, our goal here is to eat enough of 'em for fuel, but not so much that they create too much body fat. One more thing: You need fat in your diet, as I mentioned previously. But that doesn't mean you should dive into a bucket of fried chicken—you just need about 20 percent of your diet to come from fat.

Let's take a look at a couple of examples so that you can see how easy it is to work with the formulas I listed above. We'll use a 200-pound person and a 125-pound person as our guinea pigs.

200-POUND PERSON
Daily protein intake: 200 x 1 = 200 grams of protein per day
Daily carb intake: 200 x 1 = 200 grams of carbs per day
Daily fat intake: 200 x .22 = 44 grams of fat per day

125-POUND PERSON
Daily protein intake: 125 x 1 = 125 grams of protein per day
Daily carb intake: 125 x1 = 125 grams of carb per day
Daily fat intake: 125 x .22 = 28 grams of fat per day

See how easy that was? Now that you know how many grams of each nutrient you need on a daily basis, it's easy to determine how many grams of each nutrient you'll need to eat at every meal.

Step 2: Commit to Eating 4 Times a Day

Instead of eating 3 meals as you did in the Level 1 transition period, you'll eat 4 times a day in Level 2. I recommend that you eat 3 regular meals and consume 1 protein shake per day. You'll be able to fit the program into your life more easily if you can have a protein drink while you're at work or at a point in the day when you just can't eat a regular meal. Do your best to evenly spread out the meals during the waking hours of the day. This usually means that you'll be eating every 3 to 5 hours.

The importance of eating frequent, smaller meals rather than larger, infrequent feedings can't be ignored. Start with the fact that your ability to digest food is better since you're not overloading your body with too much to handle at one time. Also, by forcing your body to break down some food every couple of hours, your metabolism becomes much more active and able to burn body fat. Finally, eating protein frequently creates a situation in the body called "positive nitrogen balance," which is normally associated with the preservation or enhancement of the desirable lean muscle tissue that gives your body shape and definition.

Step 3: Determine Your Personal Meal-by-Meal Nutrient Requirements

Since you now know how many grams of each nutrient you'll be eating every day and the number of meals you'll be having in every 24-hour period, we need to determine how much you'll be eating at each meal. It's easy: Simply divide your daily gram intake for each nutrient by 4, or the number of meals you'll be eating. Let's go back to the examples we used earlier:

200-POUND PERSON
Daily protein intake (200 grams) divided by 4 = 50 grams of protein per meal
Daily carb intake (200 grams) divided by 4 = 50 grams of carbs per meal
Daily fat intake (44 grams) divided by 4 = 11 grams of fat per meal

125-POUND PERSON
Daily protein intake (125 grams) divided by 4 = 31 grams of protein per meal
Daily carb intake (125 grams) divided by 4 = 31 grams of carbs per meal
Daily fat intake (28 grams) divided by 4 = 7 grams of fat per meal

Step 4: Time to Pick Your Meals

Now that you know your personal nutrient requirements for each meal, it's time to actually choose the foods you'll be eating. The great thing about this program is that you can eat the same food every day or not eat the same meal for a month—you decide how much variety you want in your meal plan. You get to choose the foods you're going to be eating from healthy, normal, everyday foods that can be found in every supermarket in the world (and restaurants, too).

I don't believe in prepackaged foods that are full of preservatives or chemicals. Do you want to eat that stuff for the rest of your life? I didn't think so. With The TRUTH program, *you're* in control of your life and you choose what goes in your mouth.

Here's how it works: If you're supposed to eat 50 grams of protein per meal, simply go to Chapter 13 and choose the protein source you want to eat. Chicken would be a good choice here, as it has about 8 grams of protein per cooked ounce. So, if you eat 6 ounces of chicken, your protein requirement is taken care of for that meal. (I know that's really 48 grams of protein, not 50—but you don't have to be exact. Just make sure that you're within a couple of grams and you'll be fine.) You'll also need to get in your 50 grams of carbs per meal. If you're in the mood for a sweet potato, I've got good news for you: One cup has 48 grams of carbohydrates, so that will certainly satisfy your carb needs for that meal. And don't forget that you need to have a little fat, too—about 11 grams. I love peanut butter, and as you'll find out, 1 tablespoon has 8 grams of fat. So 1½ tablespoons of peanut butter will give you 12 grams of fat. Now, your meal is not only tasty and satisfying, but it's also complete.

Let's go back to our previous examples to further illustrate how to create a custom meal plan that will fit your needs. (These are just samples that I'm concocting, so feel free to choose the foods you want to eat based on your own preferences and your convenience. The complete list is in the next chapter.)

Step 5: More Cheat Meals

At Level 2, you're allowed to have a cheat meal every fifth day, instead of every seventh day as you did at Level 1. At this point, I'm also hoping that you're putting more into your strength training and cardio so that we can keep revving your metabolism up to function at faster levels.

200-POUND PERSON
MEAL BREAKDOWN

Protein: 50 grams

Carbs: 50 grams

Fat: 11 grams

Meal 1

Protein: 4 egg-white omelette with 4 oz. of chicken breast = 44 grams

Carbs: 1 cup oatmeal with 3 tbsp. raisins = 50 grams

Fat: 1½ tbsp. peanut butter = 12 grams

Meal 2

Protein: 6 oz. turkey breast = 48 grams

Carbs: 2 slices rye bread and 1 medium apple = 54 grams

Fat: 1 tbsp. almond butter = 10 grams

Meal 3

Protein: 6 oz. chicken breast = 48 grams

Carbs: 1 cup baked sweet potato = 50 grams

Fat: 1½ tbsp. peanut butter = 12 grams

Meal 4

Protein: MET-Rx or any other protein powder = 50 grams

Carbs: 8 oz. pineapple juice and 2 rice cakes = 50 grams

Fat: .7 oz. peanuts = 10 grams

125-POUND PERSON
MEAL BREAKDOWN

Protein: 31 grams

Carbs: 31 grams

Fat: 7 grams

Meal 1

Protein: Protein powder = 30 grams

Carbs: 1 cup of oatmeal with 1 cup strawberries = 32 grams

Fat: 1 tbsp. peanut butter = 8 grams

Meal 2

Protein: 4 oz. turkey breast = 32 grams

Carbs: 2 slices rye bread = 32 grams

Fat: .5 oz. almonds = 8 grams

Meal 3

Protein: 4 oz. chicken breast = 32 grams

Carbs: ½ cup rice = 25 grams

Fat: .5 oz. cashew butter = 7 grams

Meal 4

Protein: 4 oz. halibut = 28 grams

Carbs: 1 cup lettuce and 1 cup broccoli with 2 tbsp.
    fat-free dressing = 30 grams

Fat: 2 oz. olives = 8 grams

*L*evel 3: Advanced Eating

This level is designed for those people who have come to The TRUTH as advanced fitness enthusiasts or for those of you who are now training at Level 3 or above. As you'll see from the food formulas below, you'll be eating more protein and slightly less fat than you did at Level 2— now that you're training harder in the gym, your body needs more protein to rebuild and repair your lean muscle tissue, and you won't need quite as much fat.

Here we go!

Step 1: Determine Your Personal Daily Nutrient Requirements

Just as you did at Level 2, the first step in creating your personalized eating plan at Level 3 is to determine the appropriate daily amount you'll need of each of the major nutrients. As you'll see, the formulas have changed a bit, but it's still extremely simple:

1.5 grams of protein per body weight
1 gram of carbohydrates per body weight
.20 grams of fat x body weight

Again, let's use our 200- and 125-pound people as examples, so you can see how these particular formulas work:

200-POUND PERSON
Daily protein intake: 200 x 1.5 = 300 grams of protein per day
Daily carb intake: 200 x 1 = 200 grams of carbs per day
Daily fat intake: 200 x .20 = 40 grams of fat per day

125-POUND PERSON
Daily protein intake: 125 x 1.5 = 187 grams of protein per day
Daily carb intake: 125 x1 = 125 grams of carbs per day
Daily fat intake: 125 x .20 = 25 grams of fat per day

Step 2: Commit to Eating 5 Times a Day

We've already discussed the value of eating smaller, frequent meals throughout the day. Here we're spreading your food out over 5 meals because otherwise your body would have a very hard time properly digesting and using the higher amounts of protein and carbs that you'll be eating at this level.

I recommend that you eat 3 regular meals and then drink 2 protein shakes per day. Do your best to evenly spread the 5 meals out throughout the waking hours of the day. This usually means that you're going to eat every 3 to 4 hours.

Step 3: Determine Your Personal Meal-by-Meal Nutrient Requirements

We've already figured out your daily nutrient consumption, and we know that you'll be eating 5 times per day, so this step is easy. Simply divide your daily gram intake for each nutrient by 5 to get the nutrient breakdown for each of your daily meals. Now, let's go back to the examples we used earlier.

200-POUND PERSON

Daily protein intake (300 grams) divided by 5 = 60 grams of protein per meal
Daily carb intake (200 grams) divided by 5 = 40 grams of carbs per meal
Daily fat intake (40 grams) divided by 5 = 8 grams of fat per meal

125-POUND PERSON

Daily protein intake (187 grams) divided by 5 = 37 grams of protein per meal
Daily carb intake (125 grams) divided by 5 = 25 grams of carbs per meal
Daily fat intake (25 grams) divided by 5 = 5 grams of fat per meal

Step 4: Time to Pick Your Meals

Just like in Level 2, your next step is to choose the foods you'll be eating from the list in the next chapter. Again, you can eat the same food every day or not eat the same meal for months.

Step 5: More Cheat Meals

At Level 3, you're allowed to have 2 cheat meals per week, separated by at least 3 days. At this point, I hope that you're putting more into your workouts so that we can keep that metabolism functioning at an even higher level.

Let's go back to our examples to see how to create a custom meal plan that will fit your needs.

200-POUND PERSON MEAL BREAKDOWN

Protein: 60 grams

Carbs: 40 grams

Fat: 8 grams

Meal 1
Protein: 6 egg-white omelette with 5 oz. of chicken breast = 58 grams
Carbs: 1 cup oatmeal with 2 tbsp. raisins = 43 grams
Fat: 1 tbsp. peanut butter = 8 grams

Meal 2
Protein: 7 oz. turkey breast = 56 grams
Carbs: 2 slices rye bread and 2 apricots = 40 grams
Fat: .5 oz. almonds = 8 grams

Meal 3
Protein: MET-Rx or any protein powder = 60 grams
Carbs: 1 cup banana and strawberries = 40 grams
Fat: .6 oz. peanuts = 8 grams

Meal 4
Protein: 7 oz. chicken breast = 56 grams
Carbs: ¾ cup baked sweet potato = 37.5 grams
Fat: 1 tbsp. peanut butter = 8 grams

Meal 5
Protein: Protein powder = 60 grams
Carbs: 8 oz. pineapple juice and 1 rice cake = 30 grams
Fat: .6 oz. peanuts = 8 grams

125-POUND PERSON
MEAL BREAKDOWN

Protein: 37 grams

Carbs: 25 grams

Fat: 5 grams

Meal 1
Protein: MET-Rx or any protein powder = 37 grams
Carbs: 1 cup oatmeal = 25 grams
Fat: ½ tbsp. peanut butter = 4 grams

Meal 2
Protein: 4 oz. turkey breast = 32 grams
Carbs: 2 slices rye bread = 32 grams
Fat: .33 oz. peanuts = 4 grams

Meal 3
Protein: 4.5 oz. chicken breast = 36 grams
Carbs: ½ cup rice = 25 grams
Fat: .25 oz. cashews = 3.5 grams

Meal 4
Protein: MET-Rx or any protein powder = 37 grams
Carbs: 1 cup of oatmeal = 27 grams
Fat: ½ tbsp. peanut butter = 4 grams

Meal 5
Protein: 5 oz. halibut = 36 grams
Carbs: 1 cup lettuce and 1 cup broccoli with
    2 tbsp. fat-free dressing = 30 grams
Fat: 2 oz. olives = 8 grams

A Few Lingering Questions

As you read through the levels of healthy eating outlined in this chapter, some questions may have occurred to you. Don't worry—I've got your answers.

"When is the best time to eat?" You should definitely start eating within an hour of waking up in the morning. You see, your metabolism was at rest for at least 6 hours while you slept, so a meal will kick start it for the day. Additionally, eating will get your energy levels up, so you'll feel upbeat and ready to tackle your day. Once you've had your first meal, eat in evenly spaced intervals to get in the appropriate number of meals for the day.

"I noticed that there aren't many dairy options on the nutrient-choice list. Why not?" It's my opinion that dairy products have a funny way of sitting on the body. Even though they're often low fat or even fat free, they seem to have a negative effect on the body's ability to shed fat. Maybe it's the sodium, or it has something to do with the chemical composition of dairy foods—I can't give you a precise scientific reason, but my observations over the years have led me to conclude that they just aren't the best choice for helping most people who want to shed pounds.

The hitch is that you need to get some calcium in your body, which you can easily do by taking a quality vitamin/mineral product. If you feel that you absolutely must eat dairy, here are a few tips: (1) Always choose low-fat or fat-free items; (2) use your cheat meal to eat your dairy; and (3) go without it when you're not on a cheat meal. Once you've reached your goal and have entered "maintenance mode," feel free to use dairy products more regularly. (**Note:** I'm not that big on soy. In new studies, it's been shown to lower testosterone levels in men and slow down the thyroid. I don't use soy, nor do I recommend it.)

"I noticed that on the food chart in the next chapter, there are fat grams in parentheses next to certain protein foods. What does this mean?" Some protein-rich foods, such as lean red meats and certain types of fish, have higher amounts of fat in them. When you eat one of those foods, you should also multiply the number in parentheses (the fat content in that serving) by the portion size and then count that in your fat intake for that meal. For example, a 1-ounce cooked serving of bass contains approximately 7 grams of protein and 1 gram of fat. Now let's say that you need to eat 50 grams of protein and 11 grams of fat per meal—you'd eat 7 ounces of bass, which would yield 40 grams of protein and 7 grams of fat. You'll have met your protein requirement, and you'll have consumed 7 grams of fat. Since you were entitled to 11 grams of fat at this meal, you can take in another 4 grams (such as a half tablespoon of peanut butter) and these 2 nutrient groups will have been satisfied. The reason that only certain foods have both protein and fat intake for you to factor in is that the rest of the foods have less significant amounts of fat that I don't feel will disturb the ratios of food you should be consuming.

"How long before or after I work out should I eat a meal?" This is an individual decision. Some people like to eat a few hours before they work out, and others like to eat within an hour of training. Figure out what feels best for you. However, I recommend that you start out by eating an hour or so before you train so that you'll have the energy you'll need to exercise, but don't feel too full or bloated, which could negatively affect your ability to get the most out of your workout.

After you train, you should eat a meal within an hour. There's a window of time after you work out when your body needs protein and carbohydrates to recuperate and replenish the nutrients that you've burned while you trained. If you have a hard time eating soon after you finish training, use one of your protein shakes with some delicious carbs blended in (such as bananas, frozen strawberries, or pineapple) for this meal.

In the next chapter, I've taken common foods and broken them down into an easy chart that you can use to plan your meals. Have fun with "The Big Food Chart"!

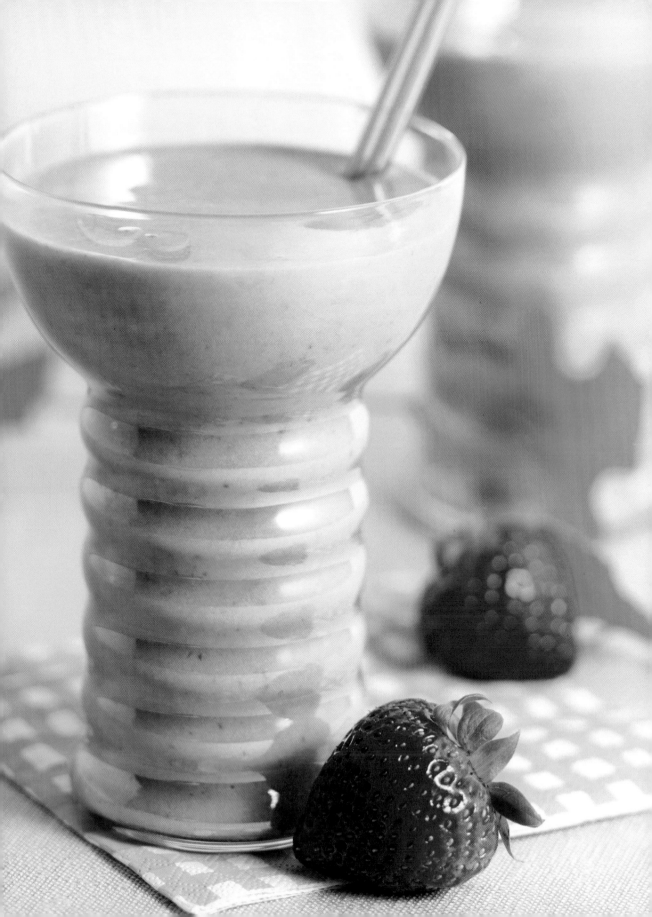

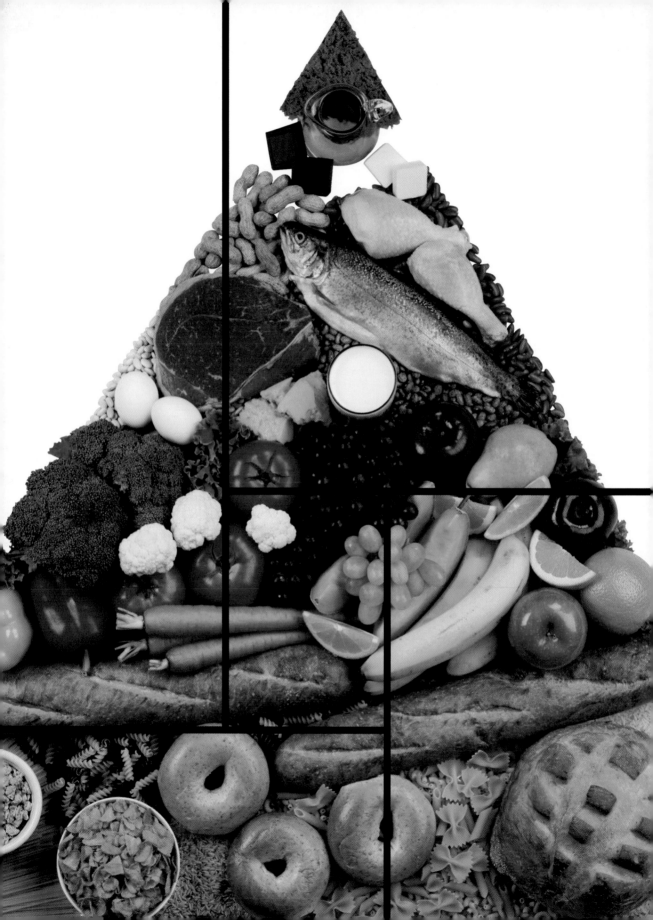

CHAPTER 12

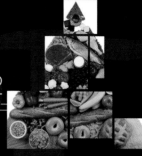

THE BIG FOOD CHART

PROTEIN SOURCES

Food	Serving Size	Protein
MEAT/EGGS		
Beef, flank steak	1 oz. raw weight	7 (3 fat)
Beef, ground	1 oz. raw weight	7 (5 fat)
Beef, top round, eye of round or full round (lean only)	1 oz. raw weight	9
Chicken breast, boneless	1 oz. cooked weight	8
Cottage cheese, fat-free	½ cup	7
Egg substitute	¼ cup	6
Egg white	1 large	3
Protein powder, such as MET-Rx Protein Plus	1 scoop	16
Turkey breast, boneless	1 oz. cooked weight	8
Veal (lean only) braised or stewed	1 oz. cooked weight	10
FISH/SEAFOOD		
Bass	1 oz. cooked weight	7 (1 fat)
Clams	1 oz. cooked weight (meat only)	7 (1 fat)
Cod	1 oz. cooked weight	6
Crab	1 oz. cooked weight (meat only)	6
Haddock	1 oz. cooked weight	7
Halibut	1 oz. cooked weight	7
Lobster	1 oz. cooked weight (meat only)	6
Orange roughy	1 oz. cooked weight	5
Salmon	1 oz. cooked weight	6 (3 fat)
Scallops	1 oz. raw weight	5
Sea bass	1 oz. cooked weight	7
Shrimp	1 oz. cooked weight	6
Snapper	1 oz. cooked weight	8
Swordfish	1 oz. cooked weight	7 (2 fat)
Trout	1 oz. cooked weight	7 (2 fat)
Tuna steak	1 oz. cooked weight	8
Tuna in water, canned and drained	1 oz. cooked weight	7
Whitefish	1 oz. cooked weight	7 (2 fat)

CARBOHYDRATE SOURCES

Food	Serving Size	Carbs
FRUIT/FRUIT JUICES		
Apple	½ medium	11
Apple juice	4 oz.	15
Apricots, dried	1 oz.	10
Apricots, fresh	3 medium	12
Banana	½ medium	14
Cantaloupe	1 cup	14
Cherries with pits	1 cup	13
Grapefruit	½ medium	11
Grapefruit juice	4 oz.	13
Grapes	1 cup	15
Kiwi	1 medium	12
Mango, peeled	2 oz.	10
Nectarine	1 medium	16
Orange	1 medium	17
Orange juice	4 oz.	14
Peach	1 medium	10
Pear	½ medium	13
Pineapple	½ cup	10
Pineapple juice	4 oz.	15
Plum	1 medium	9
Raisins	2 tbsp.	16
Strawberries	½ cup	6
Watermelon	1 cup	12
BREADS		
Bagel	1 large	43
Pita bread, white	1 slice	29
Pumpernickel bread	1 slice	16
Rye bread	1 slice	16
Wheat bread	1 slice	12
CEREALS/GRAINS		
Cream of Wheat	1 cup	30
Grape-Nuts	1 oz.	24
Nutri-Grain	¾ cup	24

CARBOHYDRATE SOURCES (cont.)

Food	Serving Size	Carbs
Oatmeal	1/2 cup dry weight	27
Puffed wheat	1 cup	11
Shredded Wheat	1 piece	19
PASTA/POTATOES/RICE		
Pasta, various types	1 oz. uncooked	21
Potato, baked	1/2 medium	26
Potato, boiled	1 medium, peeled	27
Potato, sweet	1/2 cup baked	25
Rice, brown	1/2 cup cooked	25
Rice, white	1/2 cup cooked	25
Rice, white (instant)	1/2 cup cooked	20
Rice cakes	1 regular	9
Yam	1/2 cup boiled or baked	19
VEGETABLES		
Asparagus	1 cup or 12 spears	9
Beans, green	1/2 cup raw, boiled, or canned	4
Beets, sliced	1/2 cup boiled	9
Broccoli	1 cup cooked	10
Brussels sprouts	1 cup cooked	13
Cabbage	1 cup cooked	7
Carrots	1/2 cup or 1 whole raw	8
Cauliflower	1 cup cooked or raw	6
Celery	1 cup or 4 stalks	4
Corn	1/4 cup cooked	7
Cucumber	2 cups	6
Eggplant	1 cup cooked	6
Lentils	1/4 cup cooked or dry	10
Lettuce, iceberg	1/2 head	6
Lettuce, romaine	3 cups	4
Mushrooms (cooked)	1 cup	8
Mushrooms (raw)	1 cup	3
Onions	1/2 cup raw	6
Peas	1/2 cup cooked or dry	6
Peppers, green	1 pepper	4

Peppers, red	1 pepper	4
Radishes	4 medium	1
Sauerkraut	1 cup canned	10
Spinach	1 cup cooked	7
Tomatoes	1 raw	5
Squash, summer	1 cup cooked	8
Squash, winter	½ cup baked	9

FAT SOURCES

Food	Serving Size	Fat
NUTS/NUT BUTTERS		
Almonds	½ oz.	8
Almond butter	½ oz.	8
Cashews	½ oz.	7
Cashew butter	½ oz.	7
Macadamia nuts	¼ oz.	6
Peanuts	½ oz.	7
Peanut butter	1 tbsp.	8
Walnuts	½ oz.	8
OILS		
Oil, almond	1 tsp.	5
Oil, canola	1 tsp.	5
Oil, corn	1 tsp.	5
Oil, olive	1 tsp.	5
Oil, peanut	1 tsp.	5
Oil, sesame	1 tsp.	5
OTHER		
Avocado	1 oz. trimmed	5
Guacamole	1 tbsp.	6
Olives	1 oz. green, pitted	4

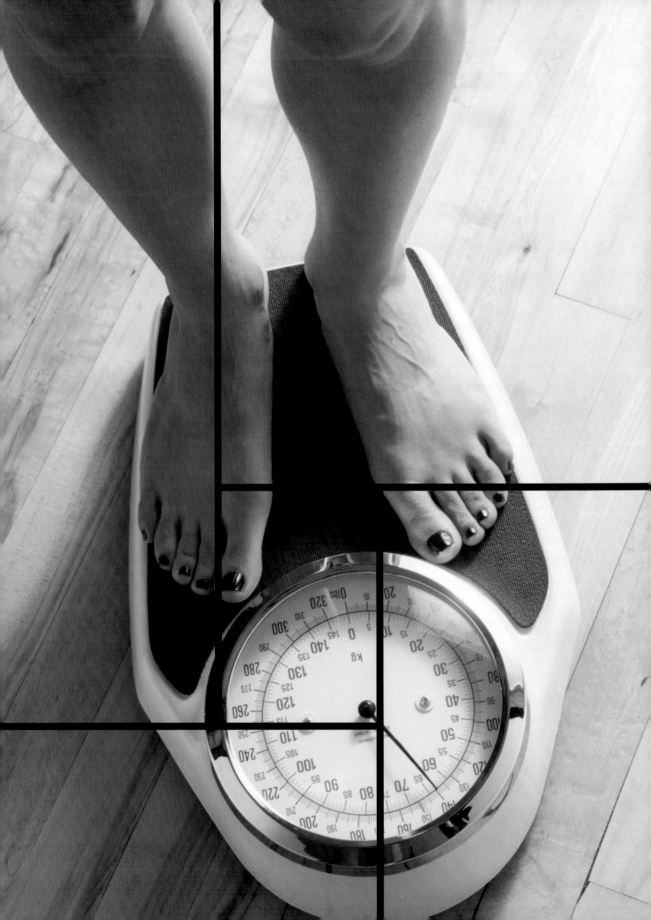

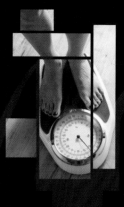

CHAPTER 13

WHAT I DO

The number-one question tossed my way is: "Frank, what exactly do *you* do to stay in shape?" I offer a few of my favorite programs in this chapter, but I want you to understand that your body is different from mine. What I do works for me—and hopefully, by now you've found The TRUTH for *your* body.

Having said that, here are the diets that have been most effective for me over the years:

CURRENT DIET PLAN (ORDINARY DAY)

Meal 1: Eggs, turkey sausage, oatmeal, coffee

Meal 2: MET-Rx protein powder mixed with water*

Meal 3: Chicken, potato, vegetables, salad

Meal 4: MET-Rx protein powder mixed with water

Meal 5: Turkey, pasta, vegetables, salad

Note: I drink 8–10 glasses of water a day and use olive oil on my salad for extra fat.

*Substitute MET-Rx protein bar for shake

BODYBUILDING DIET, PRE-CONTEST (1996)

Meal 1: 12 egg whites, half a bowl of oatmeal

Meal 2: MET-Rx original drink mix

Meal 3: 16 oz. chicken breast, small potato

Meal 4: MET-Rx original drink mix

Meal 5: 16 oz. lean beef, small potato

Meal 6: MET-Rx original drink mix

BODYBUILDING DIET, OFF-SEASON

Meal 1: 12 egg whites, 6 pancakes, 1 banana

Meal 2: MET-Rx shake, tuna sandwich

Meal 3: 16 oz. beef, pasta, vegetables

Meal 4: MET-Rx shake, bowl of rice

Meal 5: 16 oz. turkey, pasta, vegetables

Meal 6: MET-RX shake, bowl of rice

Meal 7: Whatever I wanted to eat, I ate!

MY ALL-TIME FAVORITE HEALTHY SNACKS

Rice cakes with hummus or natural peanut butter

Air-popped popcorn with butter substitute

No-sugar/low-carbohydrate frozen yogurt

Salsa on mini whole-wheat pita bread

Peanut butter, light Cool Whip, and low-fat chocolate pop mixed together—YUM!

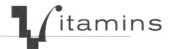itamins

It seems as if almost every store has thousands of bottles of vitamins for sale. Which ones should you take, and how much? Are they safe? There are lots of legitimate vitamin and mineral supplements on the market that deliver what they promise, but there are also many that are a total waste of money. If I were to address each and every supplemental product that's out there, this book would be 5,000 pages long. So my advice to anyone who purchases a vitamin, mineral, or sports supplement is: Research that product before you ingest it. Ask your doctor or an herbalist or purchase a book on the subject.

Everyone's body has different supplemental needs, which are based on numerous factors such as age, weight, gender, and health and fitness needs. Giving everyone the same supplemental program would be a waste of time, but I do believe that you should take vitamin, mineral, and sport supplements because they'll give your body numerous benefits. Just be smart in choosing the ones you take.

Following is what I take on an ordinary day. I may introduce a new supplement or nutritional product into this equation—it all depends on my needs and goals. (Once again, remember that this works for *my* body):

MY PERSONAL SUPPLEMENT LIST

Vitamin C

Vitamin E

B-complex

Fiber supplement

Multimineral supplement

Calcium

Saw palmetto

Papaya enzyme

Met-Rx (Ready to Drink) 40®

Met-Rx Original Drink Mix® in chocolate or vanilla

Met-Rx Protein Plus Bars®

Weight Training

I believe that life is a learning process, and the best way to learn something is to simply do it. It follows that the last 20 years have been a great learning experience for me. In that time, I've tried hundreds of weight-training routines and logged thousands of hours in the gym. I wish I could have told you in the first chapter that I was just born with this body and spend all my time in a La-Z-Boy, but *nobody's* that lucky. It's taken me a very long time to go from tall, skinny "Frankenstein" to the man I am today, with a body I'm proud to call my own. Am I happy with myself? Please. I still see room for improvement, and I continue to work just as hard in the gym as I did when I was that kid from Queens who desperately wanted to add some muscle to his scrawny frame. But these days my goals are much different than they were 10, 5, or even 3 years ago. I now train for the following reasons: (1) because I love it; (2) for my health; and (3) to achieve the best body I can.

I think it's important for people who read this book to know what kind of training routine I follow on a daily basis—after all, I follow The TRUTH, too. I do Level 4 exercises and mix in advanced techniques from Level 5. After all the years I've spent in the gym and all the different workouts I've followed, this is without a doubt the most effective plan for me.

My typical weight-training day goes like this: I get up early in the morning, eat breakfast, shower, and head to the gym. I start my day by training 2 clients before I start my own routine because I've learned that training other people motivates me. I know that when I get to the gym there's someone waiting and counting on me to make them a healthier person. They have confidence in my abilities to get them in shape and they do everything they can in that session to perform the workout plan I've given them. Their enthusiasm and determination to succeed has a major effect and rubs off on me.

By this time, I'm ready to train. Everyone needs motivation to succeed, so I use my clients' personal goals to motivate myself, and I have a training partner who pushes me throughout my workout. I've trained with countless people in my lifetime, and I have just one thing to say about finding a training partner: Be very careful. For every fantastic training partner, you'll find 100 horrible ones. The last thing you need is someone bringing you down during your workouts by telling you their problems. Don't let anybody keep you from succeeding by being late, talking during your set, or failing to follow your personal program. The gym is about one thing only—it's your time to work on you.

Even though I have a great training partner, I do train on my own at least 30% of the time because of conflicting schedules and my frequent traveling. Here's how I get my mind ready for my workout: I put on some music and proceed to warm up. (As an aside, I like all types of music while training. I listen to techno when I do cardio, hard rock when I weight-train, and alternative when I do my stretching or yoga.) Next I do a 5-minute warm-up on the bike followed by a full-body stretch. After grabbing my water, towel, and training log, I'm ready to train. I'm warmed up and motivated, and my mind is ready to focus on my training session.

As I mentioned before, I use my Level 4 training program, plus I incorporate advanced techniques from Level 5 to make my workout more challenging and productive. There are no secret exercises, no great feats of strength, and no surprises. The reason I'm maybe a little further along in the game than you are is because I've been training nearly my entire life. Some of you will pass right by me as you continue on the program; but remember, *consistency is key.* I want you to keep in mind that weight training should always be a part of your life.

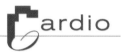

ardio

When I started lifting weights, I'd rarely, if ever, use the exercise bike or run on the treadmill. I really didn't know much about cardiovascular exercise and didn't really care. The only thing I was interested in was packing on the muscle. I didn't want to lose any of that hard-earned brawn I'd put on, so cardio was like Kryptonite to my mind. I soon learned how wrong I was—doing cardio actually ended up enhancing my physique . . . and my health.

Now I do some sort of cardio activity a minimum of 5 days a week. Some weeks I do it more, but never less. Besides running, biking, and using an elliptical trainer, I like to add kickboxing, basketball, golf, and other activities to my program. Notice that I said "add," not "substitute." And I always have four things with me for my cardio workout: water, a towel, my training log, and my personal CD player. Music helps me stay motivated and keeps my adrenaline flowing.

My personal cardio program varies from day to day, but the following is a sample week.

CARDIO WORKOUT

Monday: 45 minutes on an elliptical trainer at 60–70% MHR

Tuesday: 60 minutes of jogging—interval training

Wednesday: 21 minutes of running—interval training

Thursday: 60 minutes of jogging—interval training

Friday: 45 minutes of bicycling at 60–70% MHR

ADDITIONAL ACTIVITIES

Saturday: Kickboxing—sparring drills

Wednesday: Kickboxing—form, one-on-one

Friday: Bikram yoga—26 postures

The Future

I find it funny when people come up to me and say, "Hey, Frank, you look good now, but you can't keep this up forever." Why the hell not? We've got to forget the notion that weight training, cardio, and proper eating are quick fixes. Being in shape is a lifestyle, one that I plan to follow until the day I die. After all, it takes me just 2 hours a day to train, and it's easy to watch what I eat because it's my routine. I know that when I'm 70, I'll still be training because I love it so much. Of course, there may come a time when I have to adjust my workout because of my age or fitness level. I'll do so gladly, but you'll always find me in that gym. It's in my blood . . . and hopefully it's in yours now, too.

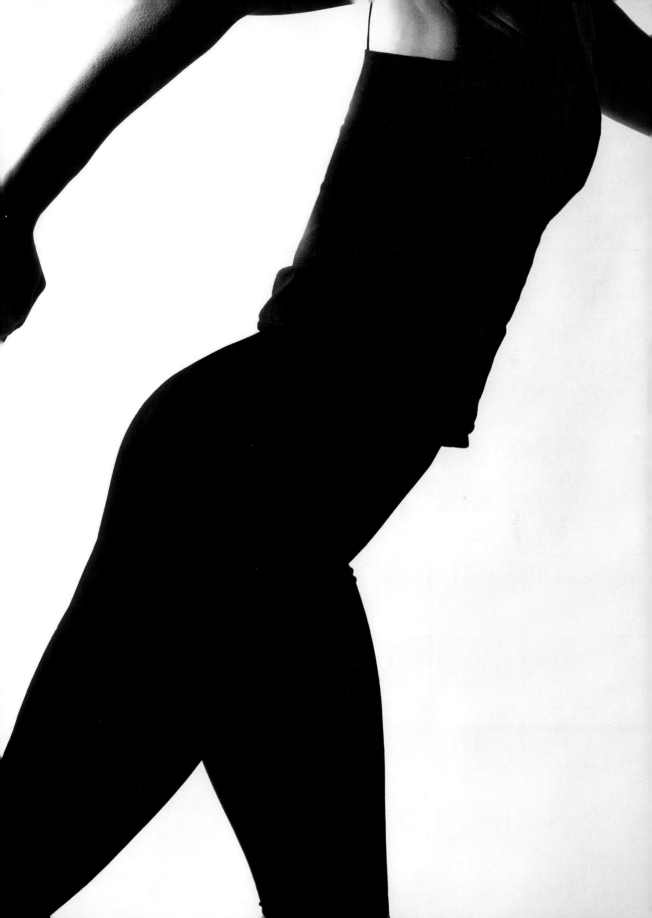

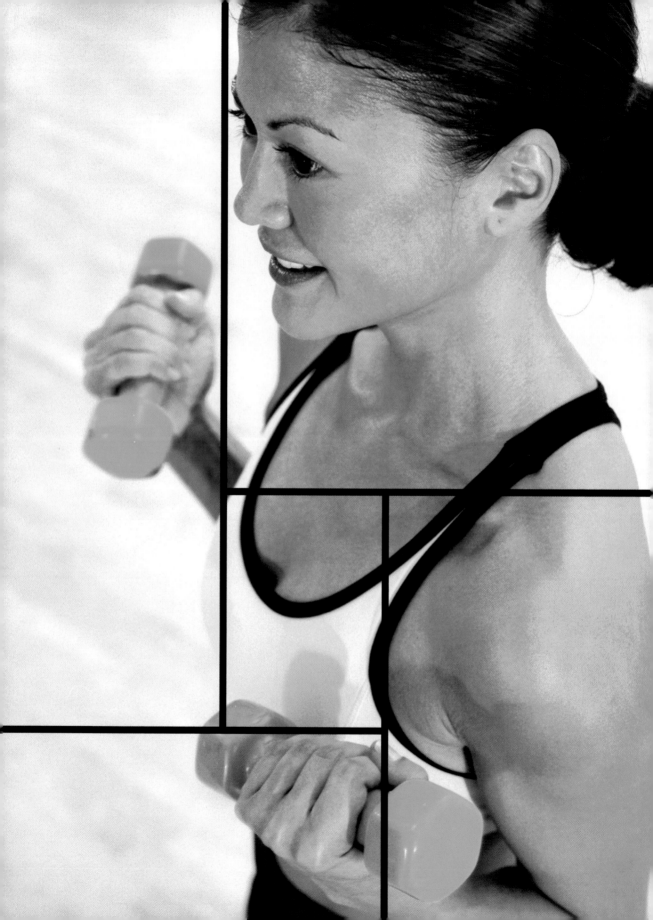

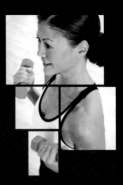

AFTERWORD

A FEW FINAL THOUGHTS FROM THOSE WHO FOUND THE TRUTH

A big fear of mine is that someone will read this book and not follow through on the plan—and thus fail to meet their particular physical and mental goals. If this happens to you—that is, if you feel like quitting—please hear my voice saying these words: "Everything worth having in life takes time and effort. You're not going to erase all of your physical and mental challenges in a short period of time. You have to stay consistent and embrace this program as your new lifestyle."

In other words, you have to say good-bye to the old you. All that time you spent eating poorly, not exercising properly, or doing anything else that didn't bring out the best in you is finally over.

Every move you make, every second you spend doing cardio, every weight you lift, and every bite of good food you put in your mouth is inching you toward the best you. Before you know it, the day will arrive when you've reached your ultimate goal. Remember that *every* step you take is a step in the right direction.

It's time to change your life. You can do it—and that's The TRUTH.

A Few Words from Some Real People

I honestly believe that hearing that others have been where you are right now and have jumped over the same hurdles you're facing will help you on the road to success. Reading their stories can only motivate you and inspire you, which is why I went to a few of my clients and told them that I was writing this book. I think it's really brave of them to share parts of their lives with everyone else, but they all did it because someone else once inspired them.

The following people used The TRUTH program to find their true selves. The stories they tell are real, honest, and in their own words. I purposefully picked an eclectic mix for this last chapter to prove that this program is for everyone—including you!

[**Editor's note:** All stories have been edited for space and clarity.]

Stephan McGrath

How did I let it get so bad? I kept asking myself.

For most of my life I've been overweight. I was a heavy child, at the mercy of classmates who reminded me of my weight on a continual basis. After eight years of constant torment, I developed a very warped body image. I was extremely self-conscious, shy, and distrustful of people. I was afraid to meet new people because I always felt that they were going to make fun of me.

By the time I entered high school, I went to the other extreme. I was never going to let people make fun of my weight again, so I embarked on a dangerous path that helped me lose a lot of weight—I just stopped eating. If I ate one meal a day, I considered it too much food. Throughout high school I was very thin, but I strangely believed that I was still fat. I often wondered if I had an eating disorder. I'm not sure I could define it in those terms—I just knew that for my entire life, food had been the enemy.

My college years were a huge struggle. Although I was approaching a "normal" weight for my height, I still suffered from my unhealthy body image and viewed myself as fat. I thought the world saw the same thing, so I joined a gym but never stuck with it. I'd go for about two months, then stop; go back three months later, train for about a week, and then stop for six months. And my idea of dieting was still "If I don't eat, I won't gain weight."

After college, the battle was completely lost. My weight fluctuated wildly—I'd lose 20 pounds but gain 25, as I continued my start-stop relationship with the gym. I was miserable, embarrassed, and afraid of running into people I hadn't seen in ages. I'd go to bars with my friends, only to stand in the corner because I thought no one would want to talk to "the fat guy."

When I turned 30, I had one of those moments that made me realize things needed to change. I was getting ready for work when I realized that I had nothing to wear. All of the clothes that

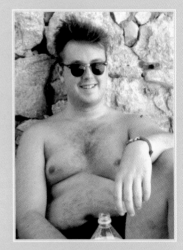

BEFORE

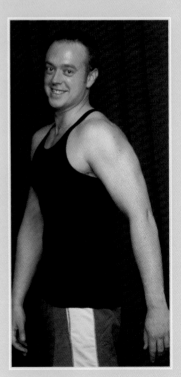

AFTER

I could comfortably fit into were in the wash. I was tired of the weight. I was tired of fighting. I was going to do things differently this time. That day, I met Frank.

When I arrived at the gym, I signed up for a trainer. I wanted someone to show me how to work out properly and how to diet. What Frank told me was completely contrary to what I thought I needed to do. It turns out that I didn't need to go to the gym three hours a day. But by the same token, I couldn't have the "perfectly sculpted" body after four weeks like they advertised in magazines. Most of all, I found out that I'd have to stop "dieting" and start eating more. Yet I'd have to choose better and healthier foods.

It was the first time that someone had actually told me the truth about eating and working out. I'll always remember Frank telling me, "You can't undo 30 years of neglect in four weeks." He definitely had my attention.

That was a year and a half ago. In that time, I've dropped more than 60 pounds, gone down four sizes, and completely changed my outlook. For the first time in my life, I'm not embarrassed of my body—no longer am I hiding it under layers of clothes. My confidence has soared, and my weight is no longer the overriding issue in my life. I even started to enjoy going to the gym!

Today, I find it incredible that the "fat guy" is now the one being asked questions about training and healthy eating. People talk to me with that look in their eyes—that "give me the magic cure" look. But I give them what Frank taught me: The TRUTH.

———————————

Tracy Stinnett

Staying in shape year round is a tough job, but it's critical to my career. As a top model and budding actress, I guess you could say that my body is my business. I was crowned Miss Bangkok Thailand in 2002, and I've been a Hawaiian Tropic model for the past eight years, regularly appearing in magazines, calendars, and TV shows. I also make countless public appearances.

When you make your living the way I do, you always have to look your best. The competition out there is tough, and the slightest slipup can mean the difference between booking a job or not.

While I do like working out, I'm a young, outgoing woman who wants to have a balanced life. I simply don't want to spend endless hours in the gym and eat rice cakes and salad every day. I kept wishing that there was a better way, a program that would allow me to enhance my body without taking up too much of my time or making me sacrifice the other things in my life that are important to me.

As you might have guessed already, The TRUTH is that program. When I met Frank at a trade show recently, he told me about his plan and offered to let me try it out. I started seeing improvements in my body in a few short weeks. My midsection and my legs got tighter almost immediately, and the overall shape of my body improved. What woman doesn't want that? The best thing about The TRUTH is that it's so easy to do. I don't feel like I'm starving myself, which is the way many models live their lives. I'm eating healthy food, but plenty of it. And now I'm in and out of the gym in about an hour. To my delight, I only have to work out four days a week, so my weekends are free. I'm really happy to have finally found a program that works, one I can stay committed to for the rest of my life.

I know my career is in better shape thanks to The TRUTH— and so is my body!

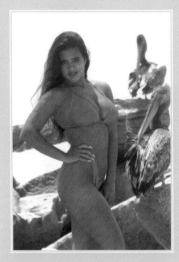

BEFORE

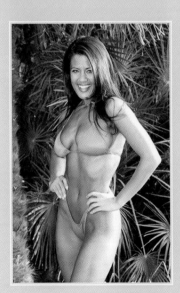

AFTER

Larry Pepe

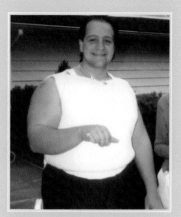

BEFORE

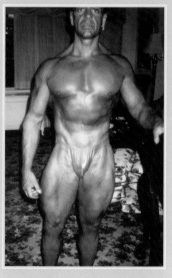

AFTER

My story is a bit different from the other success stories you'll read in this book. Unlike the scores of people who have been, and will be, fortunate enough to receive The TRUTH program in the well-written, organized, step-by-step format that you hold in your hands, I've spent the last 15 years living and experimenting with the principles that are contained in the pages of Frank's book.

Frank and I met more than a decade ago at a New York gym. His potential as a bodybuilder was obvious to anyone with an eye for a good physique. As for me, when I was in my early 20s I was clinically obese (as you can plainly see from my "before" photo). It wasn't a happy place to be—after all, when you look and feel that out of shape, you miss out on a lot. At least *I* did. My self-esteem took a beating when I'd pass a mirror or have to go shopping for clothes. I just wanted to live in sweatpants.

I became a professional bodybuilder and lost (and gained) an enormous amount of weight. I zigzagged and yo-yoed from being in decent shape to getting fat: I'd lose 40 to 50 pounds for a contest and then gain 50 to 60 back in the next few months. Talk about living at extremes—try going from obese to winning a bodybuilding contest in the same year!

Finally, I decided that I had to make a change and make a consistent year-round effort to maintain a healthy, attractive physique. That commitment, and the many years of trial and error that followed, allowed me to share what I learned about my own body with Frank, along with the many other people I've been fortunate enough to come into contact with over the years.

What I love about what Frank has done with this book is the recognition of several things we've seen work over the years. I couldn't be more proud of The TRUTH program and having the opportunity to be involved with it and Frank's metamorphosis, not only as a physical being, but also as an educator. If you're wondering what this program can offer *you,* take another look at my picture. The principles embodied in *The TRUTH* allowed me to transform my body, my self-esteem, and my life. If you read it, commit to it, and follow through with it every day, then I can virtually guarantee that it will do the same for you.

Richard Jankura

Working with stallions can be a bit dangerous, but I never really thought about my lack of size as a problem. I just have one of those metabolisms that no matter how much I ate, I stayed skinny. At 128 pounds with a 28-inch waist, I was still shopping in the children's department even though I was 40 years old. A friend turned me on to Frank Sepe and his program, so I thought I'd give it a try.

I never thought it would be possible to change my body the way I have. I now have the body I desired in my 20s and 30s. It just goes to show that when you have the determination and the right fitness program, you can accomplish the impossible.

It's kind of cool being in my new "grown-up body." And, as an equestrian athlete, the extra strength helps my riding a lot. People can't believe that I've changed so drastically. I've gone from 128 to 165 pounds in a little over a year. My lifestyle is so different since I adapted The TRUTH system as part of my everyday life.

The consistent gains I've made keep me wanting more, so I plan to do this program for the rest of my days. It's truly amazing that the guys in the gym now refer to me as "jacked." That makes me laugh because it wasn't so long ago that I was hearing skinny jokes. Now I have more confidence, more self-esteem, and the rock-hard physique I always wanted. Thanks, Frank, for helping me achieve something I never thought was possible.

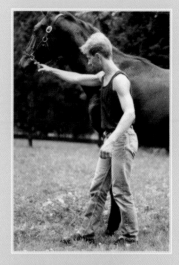

BEFORE

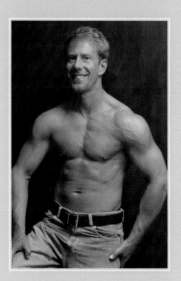

AFTER

Marilyn Groce

"You're so lucky to be thin." I hear this all the time. Trust me—luck has nothing to do with it.

The first time I started to gain weight was my senior year of high school. I went from 115 to 135 pounds, and my mom, a lifetime dieter herself, became very concerned and insisted I go on a diet. I knew absolutely nothing about nutrition, so she took me to a local clinic where they put me on pills, hormone shots, and a 500-calorie-a-day diet. I lost 20 pounds in almost no time, and left for college as skinny as a rail.

Dorm food was wall-to-wall macaroni and cheese, burgers, and fries. I ate cookies every night while I was studying, and had pizza and beer on the weekends. I never really noticed how much weight I was putting on, and by Christmas, I was 150 pounds. I was too embarrassed to go home, so I made excuses to stay at school. I kept right on eating, and by summer break I weighed 180 pounds. Now I was really fat—and I *had* to go home.

I still thought pills and starvation were the answers. I'd consume virtually no calories and then binge, and it became a vicious cycle. Soon I was up to 200 pounds and desperate. I cried all the time. I hit rock bottom when the company I worked for sent over new uniforms, and the largest one wouldn't fit me.

I tried Weight Watchers, Jenny Craig, NutriSystem, Diet Center, and Slim-Fast. I honestly don't think there's a diet out there that I haven't tried at least once. Everything worked for a while, but I always gained back the weight—plus more. I don't know how many different "diet doctors" I've gone to for pills, but soon I needed twice the recommended amount to keep my hunger under control. And in between all these "formal" programs, I tried dieting on my own, devising plans that included low calories, low carbs, and food combining. I bought every new book and tried everything my friends tried. I even tried having nothing but pre-digested liquid protein and water for six weeks—consequently, my hair started to fall out and I became dehydrated.

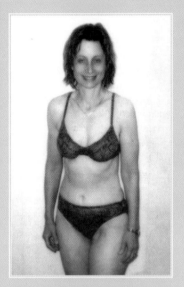

BEFORE

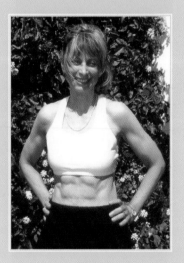

AFTER

My husband, Rod, never said anything about my weight, but he was worried about my health. My friends were concerned, and even my mom—who always wanted me thin—was scared. I remember being at a convention in San Diego and I passed out, to the point that I landed in the emergency room. Around this time, fen-phen came along, and I quickly became tolerant to it, taking six pills a day. I did that for months, until people started dying from heart-valve problems. I threw away the pills because now I was scared.

In 1998, I decided to try a different approach, so I joined a gym and hired a personal trainer. I discovered I liked it, and I even got down to 145 pounds and a size 12. Then I met Frank, who challenged me to do his program for 14 days. I thought, *What the heck?* I had nothing to lose except some pounds.

Now I'm a believer when it comes to The TRUTH. At age 54, I have the type of abs that get compliments. People always ask me, "What are you doing?" I'm not even working as hard as I've had to in the past. I looked in the mirror today (something I once tried to avoid at all costs) and wondered, *Is that the same person?* And I smile when I realized that, yes, it *is* me!

———————

K.C. Armstrong

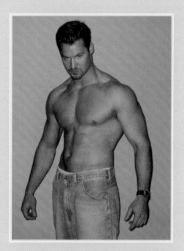

BEFORE

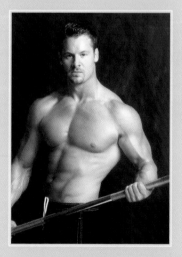

AFTER

As far back as I can remember, I've been into sports and fitness. When I was younger, I won eight wrestling championships and had a successful high school football career that led to a full scholarship to Western Kentucky University. While there, I was captain of the football team twice and was the MVP.

After I graduated, I started working full time for a top radio station in New York, WXRK 92.3, where I'm currently an associate producer. I also do stand-up comedy on the weekends at some of the Big Apple's top clubs. This hectic work schedule didn't do anything positive for my physique—not by a long shot! While I've always taken pride in my appearance and tried to stay in the best possible shape, I realized that I wasn't measuring up to the standards I've always set for myself. I wasn't necessarily fat, but I definitely wasn't happy with the way I looked or felt.

I figured that the solution would be a piece of cake: All I needed to do was to train and eat the way I used to and my body would come right back to me. It worked before, so it would have to work now. It just seemed logical to me. Sorry, K.C., no deal. After a couple of weeks and no results, I realized that my body had hit a plateau on my old program, so if I wanted to succeed, I'd need a new workout and eating plan. I bought fitness magazines and started following some of their routines. I tried one plan after the other, yet I still couldn't find a program that worked. They all looked good on paper, but when I followed them there was always a flaw. I tried no-carb diets and got uncontrollable food cravings. And the high-intensity workout program I jumped into left my joints aching after every session.

Then I met Frank Sepe. I told him about my frustrating dilemma, and he told me about the program he was developing. I decided to try The TRUTH, and the results have been fantastic. Not only does this program work and deliver great results, but I've been able to stay committed to it. Finally!

In 30 days, I made more progress than I had in the past three months! Today, my body is toned and my abs have never looked better. Let me save you all the time I wasted trying everything else under the sun before I found The TRUTH: If you want a program that's easy to follow and will give you great results if you stick with it, this is definitely the one for you. Believe me when I tell you The TRUTH works.

———————

And Finally . . .

Once again, I'd like to remind you that The TRUTH isn't a quick-fix program or a fad. It's a lifestyle and a commitment to your health, self-esteem, confidence, and most important, your happiness. You'll make consistent physical and mental improvements throughout the five phases of the program, while becoming healthier every day you stick with it.

The TRUTH isn't magic. Like anything else in life, what you get from it will equal the effort you put into it. With an honest, 100-percent commitment, you *will* find the "true you."

When I wrote this book, I hoped that it would change people's lives. Nothing makes me happier than to read the success stories that continue to pour in. Now I'd like to read yours. When you feel that you've found the true you, please send your before-and-after photos and your personal story to me at the address below. Good luck—I know you can do it!

Frank Sepe
c/o Bev Francis's Gold's Gym
235-C Robbins Lane
Syosset, NY 11791
Or you can e-mail the information to me by going to
www.FrankSepe.com and clicking on the "Success Story" link.

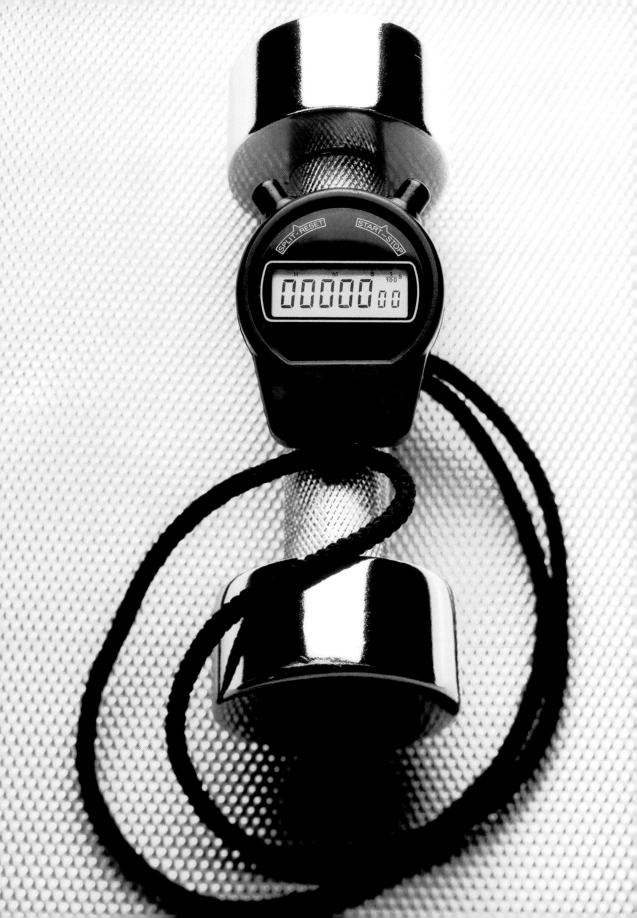

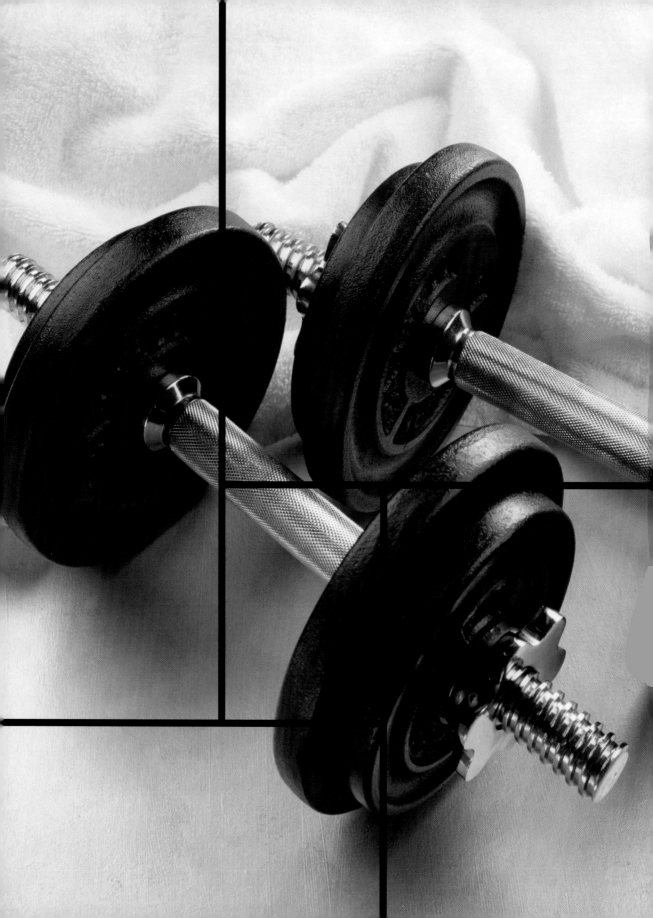

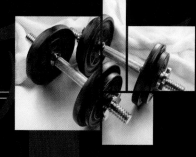

THE ACTUAL EXERCISES

This chapter includes the various exercises that we'll be doing throughout the different strength-training levels. Take a few minutes and look them over. After you've figured out which level (1–5) you're on, you'll need to come back and jot down the exercises that will take you through the next 30 days.

As you'll see, there are many variations of exercises that target the same body part. If something seems too difficult or doesn't work for you, just pick something comparable. When you're at the gym, the most important thing is to follow the instructions on proper form. It's not a race to get through your reps—instead, you need to do them correctly. I know you can do it.

As you look at the photos that accompany each exercise, I'd like you to imagine that I'm standing next to you giving you instructions. But I'm not going to wipe your sweaty brow—hey, I can only do so much in this book! So, without further ado, here are all the exercises you'll need as you finish each level. (See Chapter 7 for a complete explanation of primary versus second-

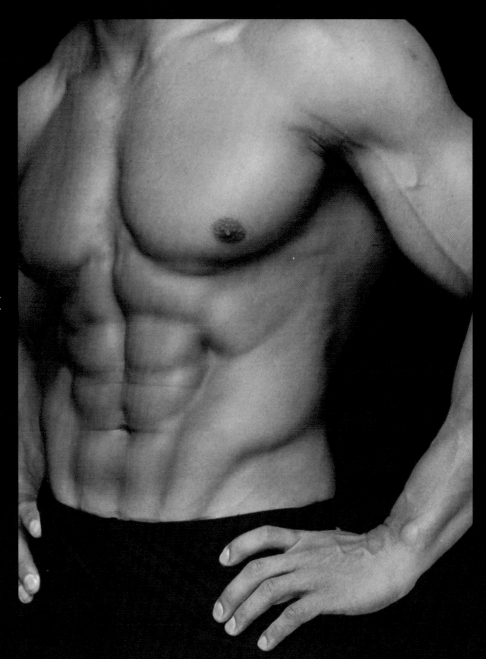

Chest

Chest

Let me get something off my chest: When I first started weight training, the only goal this 13-year-old beanpole had in mind was building a chest as well developed as his muscular dad's was. Here it is, almost two decades later, and I'm still building that perfect chest.

The good news is that exercising this area is fairly straightforward, since it's broken down into three areas: upper, middle, and lower. I strongly suggest that you work your *entire* chest in order for all of the muscle groups to be developed consistently and proportionately—this goes for men *and* women. Women, don't be afraid to do these exercises. I personally guarantee that you won't look like The Hulk in a dress.

One last note: I recommend that you don't let your ego dictate your workout. I know that men like to ask each other, "How much do you bench-press?" but don't get caught in that trap. You're in the gym to build muscle and create the body you've always wanted, not to hurt yourself in an attempt to out-bench some nimrod with an unhealthy competitive streak (and who's done so many bench presses that his pecs look like a woman's). Focus on what *you're* doing, and train smart.

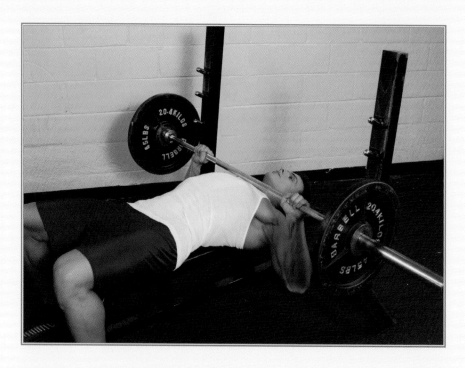

Bench Press—
Barbell

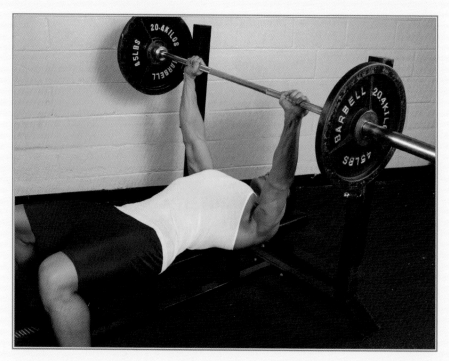

CHEST: PRIMARY EXERCISES

Bench Press—Barbell
(Targets middle, lower, and outer pectorals)

Lie on a bench with your feet flat on the floor. Grasp the bar in an overhand grip with hands shoulder-width apart. Inhale as you lift the bar off its rests and slowly lower it to mid-chest. Without resting the bar on your chest or bouncing the bar up off of it, exhale as you slowly press the bar up until your arms are fully extended (just short of locking out your elbows).

Perfect form: Keep your back flat on the bench throughout the exercise—don't arch upward.

Advanced tip: Use a grip wider than shoulder width to target the outer area of the chest.

Bench Press—
Smith Machine (Variation)
(Targets middle, lower, and outer pectorals)

Lie on a bench under a Smith machine with your feet flat on the floor. Grasp the bar with an overhand grip and hands shoulder-width apart. Inhale as you lift the bar off its rests and slowly lower it to mid-chest. Without resting the bar on your chest or bouncing the bar up off of it, exhale as you slowly press the bar up until your arms are fully extended (just short of locking out your elbows).

Perfect form: Keep your back flat on the bench throughout the exercise—don't allow it to arch upward.

Advanced tip: Use a grip wider than shoulder width to target the outer area of the chest.

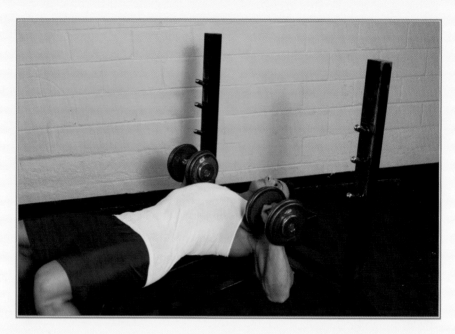

Bench Press—
Dumbbell

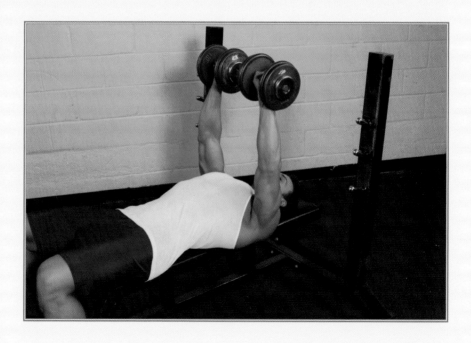

CHEST: PRIMARY EXERCISES

Bench Press–Dumbbell

(Targets middle, lower, and outer pectorals)

Sit on the end of a flat bench with your feet flat on the floor. Hold a dumbbell upright in each hand, with the weight of the dumbbell resting on your upper thighs. Lie back on the bench and tilt the dumbbells back off your thighs so that their weight is transferred to your hands. With the dumbbells held just above your chest, turn your wrists, so that instead of facing each other, your palms face toward your feet. Inhale as you slowly press the dumbbells upward and slightly toward each other until your arms are fully extended (but your elbows aren't locked). Exhale as you slowly lower the dumbbells back to just above your chest.

Perfect form: Keep your back flat on the bench throughout the exercise—don't arch upward.

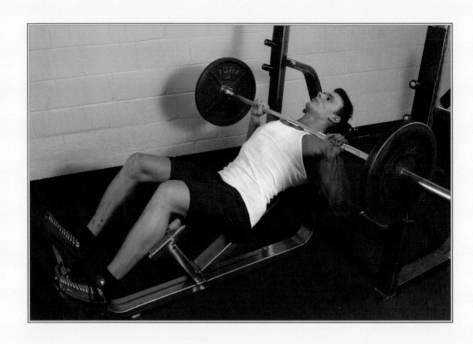

Incline Press—
Barbell

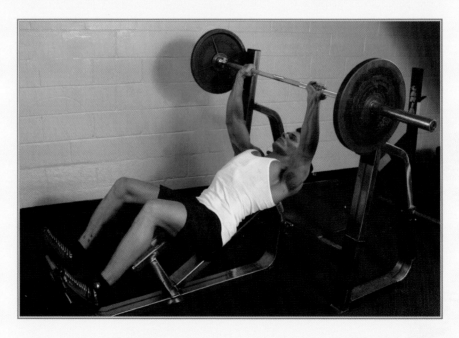

CHEST: PRIMARY EXERCISES

Incline Press–Barbell
(Targets upper-inner and medial pectorals)

Lie on an incline bench with your feet flat on the ground. Grasp the bar with an overhand grip, hands shoulder-width apart. Inhale as you lift the bar off its rests and slowly lower it to mid-chest. Without resting the bar on your chest or bouncing it off, exhale as you slowly press the bar up until your arms are fully extended (just short of locking out your elbows).

Perfect form: Keep your back flat on the bench throughout the exercise—don't allow it to arch upward.

Advanced tip: Use a grip wider than shoulder width to target the outer area of the chest.

Variation: For extra safety, especially when you don't have a spotter, use the same motion and form to do the **Incline press–Smith machine** exercise.

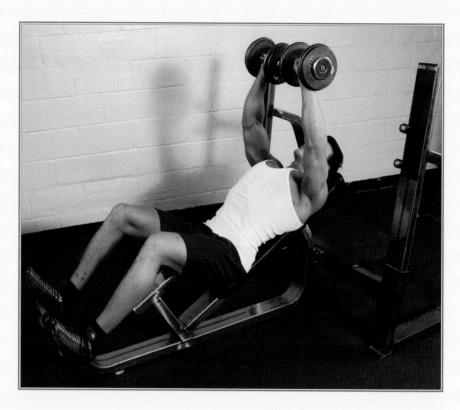

Incline Press— Dumbbell

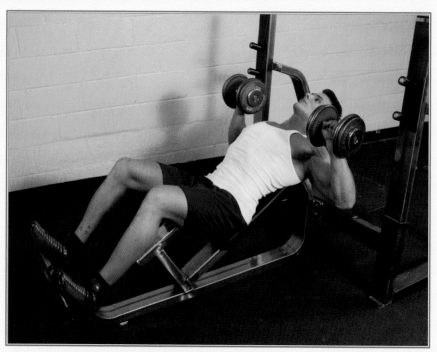

CHEST: PRIMARY EXERCISES

Incline Press—Dumbbell
(Targets upper-inner and medial pectorals)

Lie on an incline bench with your feet flat on the floor. Hold a dumbbell upright in each hand with the weight of the dumbbells resting on your thighs. Jerk the dumbbells up off your thighs and back toward your chest, moving your arms under them. Turn your wrists, so that instead of facing each other, your palms face away from you. Inhale as you slowly press the dumbbells upward and slightly toward each other until your arms are fully extended (but elbows aren't locked). Exhale as you slowly lower the dumbbells back to just above your chest.

Perfect form: Keep your back flat on the bench throughout the exercise—don't arch upward.

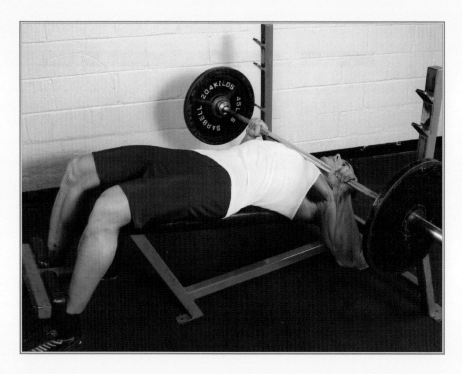

Decline Press—
Barbell

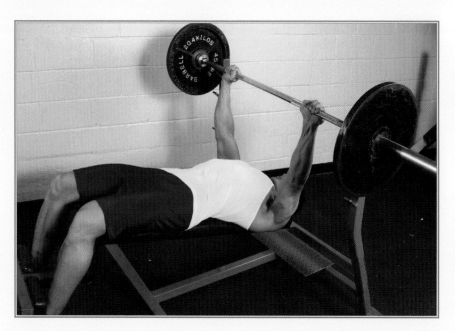

CHEST: PRIMARY EXERCISES

Decline Press—Barbell
(Targets lower-outer, upper-inner, and medial pectorals)

Lie on a decline bench with your feet firmly under the footpads. Grasp the bar in an overhand grip with hands shoulder-width apart. Inhale as you lift the bar off its rests and slowly lower it toward the lower middle part of your chest. Without resting the bar on your chest or bouncing the bar up off of it, exhale as you slowly press the bar up until your arms are fully extended (just short of locking out your elbows).

Perfect form: Keep your back flat on the bench throughout the exercise—don't allow it to arch upward.

Advanced tip: Use a grip wider than shoulder width to target the outer area of the chest.

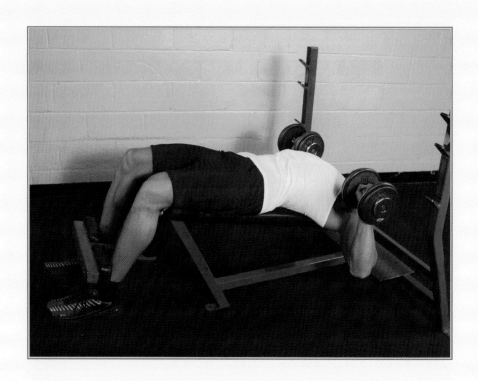

Decline Press—
Dumbbell

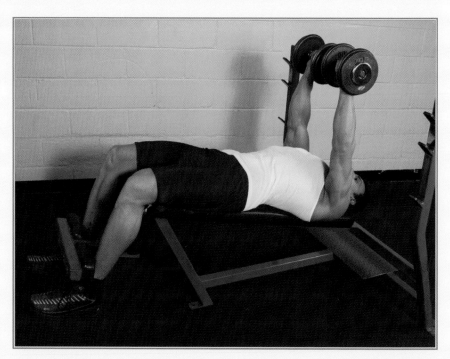

CHEST: PRIMARY EXERCISES

Decline Press—Dumbbell

(Targets lower and outer pectorals)

Sit upright on the top of a decline bench with feet under the footpads. Hold a dumbbell upright in each hand with the weight of the dumbbells resting on your thighs. Carefully recline down the bench, locking your feet under the footpads and moving the dumbbells back and down toward your chest. Turn your wrists, so that instead of facing each other, your palms face toward your feet. Inhale as you slowly press the dumbbells upward and slightly toward each other until your arms are fully extended (but elbows aren't locked). Exhale as you slowly lower the dumbbells back to just above your chest.

Perfect form: Keep your back flat on the bench throughout the exercise—don't arch upward.

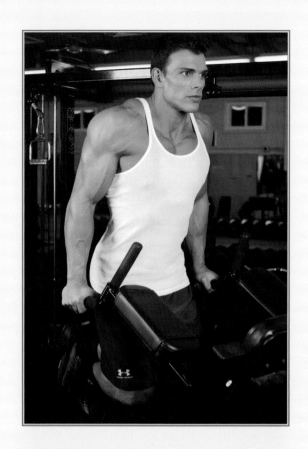

Dip—
Parellel Bars

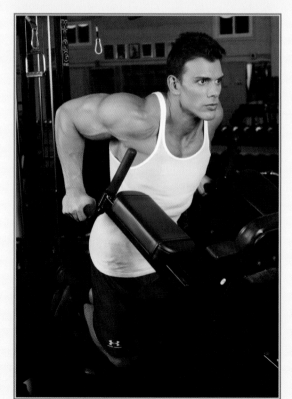

CHEST: PRIMARY EXERCISES

Dip—Parallel Bars

(Targets lower and outer pectorals)

With both hands, grasp the horizontal bars at your sides. Press your body weight up onto your arms until your hands are at waist level. Bend your knees so that your feet are well above the ground. Inhale as you slowly lower your body until your hands are just below chest height. Without bouncing, exhale as you slowly press your body back up until your hands are again at waist level (don't lock your elbows).

Perfect form: Throw your chest up and out during the entire motion, and keep your head up. Look straight ahead, not down. Slow motion is key to getting a good pump here. Keep your elbows in close to your sides.

Advanced tips: Go as low as you can to get a better chest contraction. And the difficulty of this exercise can be increased by adding weight to your weight belt.

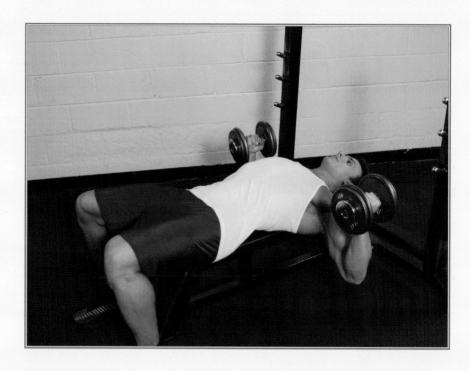

Fly—Dumbbell

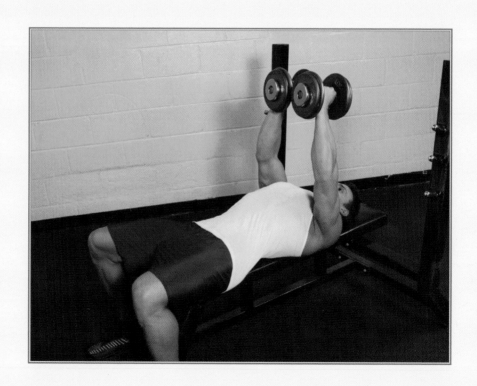

CHEST: SECONDARY EXERCISES

Fly—Dumbbell

(Targets middle, lower, and inner/outer pectorals)

Sit on the end of a flat bench with feet flat on the floor. Hold a dumbbell upright in each hand, with the weight of the dumbbells resting on your upper thighs. Lie back on the bench as you lift the dumbbells off your thighs. Press them up until they're at arm's length directly over your chest, with your elbows bent at a 10-degree angle. Turn the dumbbells so that your palms are facing each other. Maintaining the bend in your elbows, inhale as you slowly lower the dumbbells straight out to your sides, as low as you can go. Exhale as you slowly lift the dumbbells back up high over your chest.

Perfect form: The key to good flys is correct arm position. Keep your elbows bent, and think of giving someone a bear hug as you move the dumbbells through a smooth arc. Also be sure to use a weight that doesn't jeopardize your form—if you use a weight that's too heavy and you bounce it at the bottom of the exercise, you can tear your pectoral muscle. And keep your back flat on the bench.

Advanced tip: At the top of the motion, squeeze the dumbbells together so that you get a good pectoral contraction.

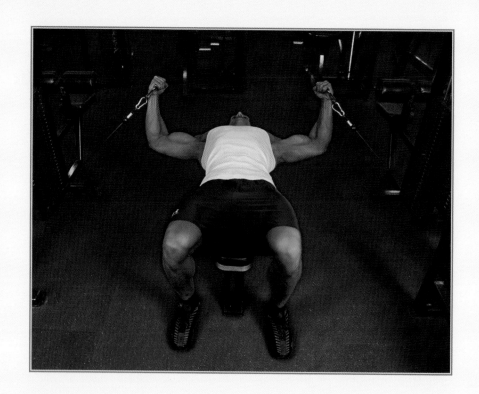

Fly—Cables
with Bench

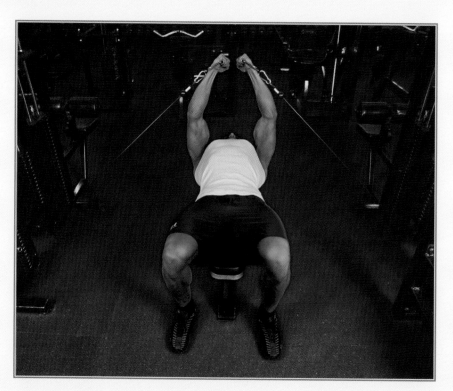

CHEST: SECONDARY EXERCISES

Fly—Cables with Bench

(Targets middle, lower, and inner/outer pectorals)

Position a flat bench between the cables on a twin-cable machine. Attach handles to each of the opposing low cables. Grasp the left handle in your left hand and the right handle in your right hand (palms facing up). Next, lie on your back with your feet flat on the floor. Pull the handles up to the starting position: arms fully extended above your chest, palms facing each other, and elbows bent at a 10-degree angle. Maintaining the bend in your elbows, inhale as you slowly lower the cables straight out to your sides, as low as you can go. Exhale as you slowly pull the handles back up to the starting position.

Perfect form: Again, the key is correct arm position: Keep your elbows bent (think *bear hug*) as you move the cables through a smooth, controlled arc. Your arms should mirror each other, moving at the same speed. Don't jerk the cables up, and keep your back flat on the bench.

Advanced tip: Focus on your contraction at the top of the movement, intensely squeezing your chest muscles for a second or two.

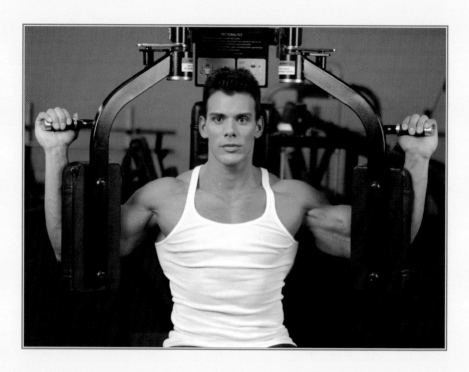

Fly—Pec Deck

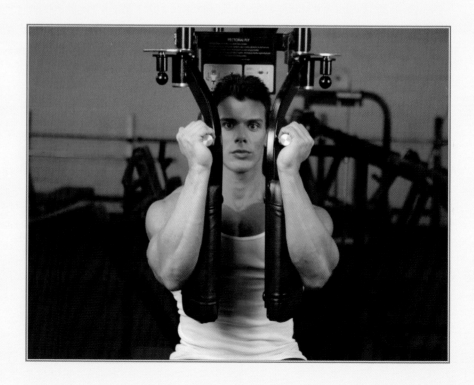

CHEST: SECONDARY EXERCISES

Fly–Pec Deck

(Targets middle and inner/outer pectorals)

Machines will vary here—some will have upright seats, some inclined—but almost every gym in America has one. Adjust the seat height so that when you grasp the handles, your upper arms form a 90-degree angle with your torso, and your elbows also form 90-degree angles. Sit down and lightly grasp the handles, your forearms firmly against the arm pads. Inhale as you slowly push with your forearms to bring the pads together in front of your chest. Squeeze your pecs hard. Then exhale as you slowly let the pads spread your arms back out to your sides, completely stretching your pecs.

Perfect form: Keep your back flat against the back pad and don't round your shoulders. Keep your hands relaxed. Don't press on the handles, which will make your forearms lift off the pads—instead, press from your elbows, keeping your forearms flat against the arm pads.

Advanced tip: Focus on getting a good stretch when your arms are spread, and a killer contraction when they're together.

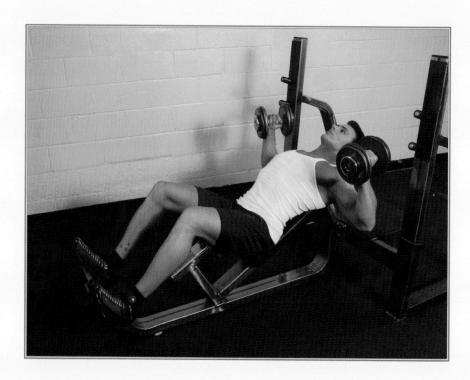

Incline Fly—
Dumbbell

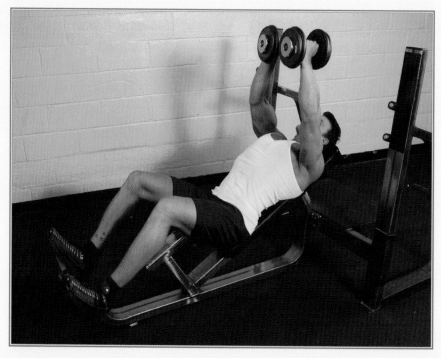

CHEST: SECONDARY EXERCISES

Incline Fly–Dumbbell

(Targets upper-inner/outer pectorals)

Sit on the edge of an incline bench with your feet flat on the floor. Hold a dumbbell upright in each hand, with the weight of the dumbbells resting on your upper thighs. Lie back on the bench as you lift the dumbbells off your thighs. Press them up until they're at arm's length directly over your chest, with your elbows bent at a 10-degree angle. Turn the dumbbells so that your palms are facing each other. Maintaining the bend in your elbows, inhale as you slowly lower the dumbbells straight out to your sides, as low as you can go. Exhale as you slowly lift the dumbbells back up high over your chest.

Perfect form: Keep your elbows bent (think *bear hug*) as you move the dumbbells through a smooth arc. Your arms should mirror each other, moving at the same speed. Keep your feet on the floor and your back against the pad. And don't arch your back.

Advanced tips: Get your elbows back as far as you can to maximize this exercise. For a better contraction, squeeze the dumbbells together and hold for two seconds at the top of the motion.

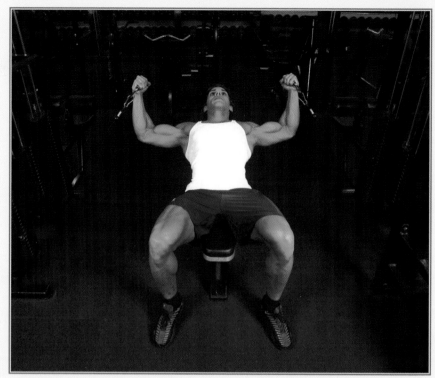

Incline Fly—
Cables

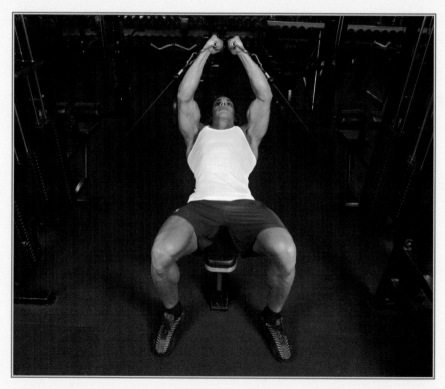

CHEST: SECONDARY EXERCISES

Incline Fly—Cables
(Targets upper-inner/outer pectorals)

Position an incline bench between the cables on a twin-cable machine. Attach handles to each of the opposing low cables. Grasp the left handle in your left hand and the right handle in your right hand (palms facing up). Lie on the bench with your feet flat on the floor, and pull the handles up to the starting position: arms fully extended above your chest, palms facing each other, and elbows bent at a 10-degree angle. Maintaining the bend in your elbows, inhale as you slowly lower the cables straight out to your sides, as low as you can go. Exhale as you slowly pull the handles back up to the starting position.

Perfect form: Keep your elbows bent (think *bear hug*) as you move the cables through a smooth, controlled arc. Your arms should mirror each other, moving at the same speed. Don't jerk the cables up, and keep your back flat on the bench.

Advanced tip: Focus on your contraction at the top of the movement, intensely squeezing your chest muscles for a second or two.

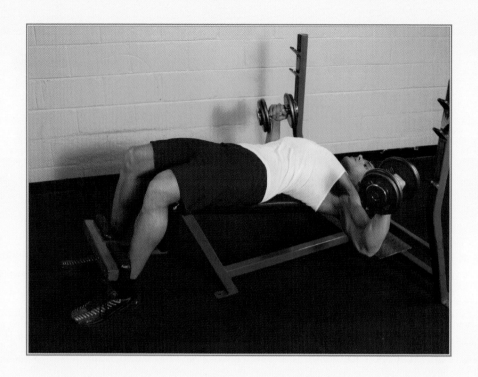

Decline Fly—
Dumbbell

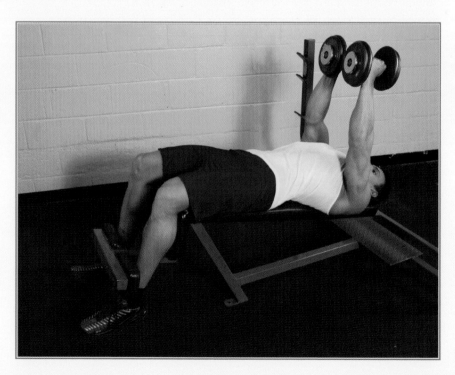

CHEST: SECONDARY EXERCISES

Decline Fly—Dumbbell
(Targets lower-inner/outer pectorals)

Sit upright on the top of a decline bench with feet under the footpads. Hold a dumbbell upright in each hand, the weight of the dumbbells resting on your thighs. Carefully recline down the bench, locking your feet under the footpads, and move the dumbbells back and down toward your chest. Press the dumbbells straight up from your chest to the starting position: arms fully extended with your palms facing each other, with a 10-degree bend in your elbows. Maintaining the bend in your elbows, inhale as you slowly lower the dumbbells straight out to your sides, as low as you can go. Exhale as you press the dumbbells back up to the starting position, contracting your pecs fully at the top.

Perfect form: Keep your elbows bent (think *bear hug*) as you move the dumbbells through a smooth, controlled arc. Your arms should mirror each other, moving at the same speed. Don't arch your back off the bench.

Advanced tips: In this position, your blood rushes to your head quickly, so don't forget to breathe. And don't bang the dumbbells together at the top—bring them together *gently*.

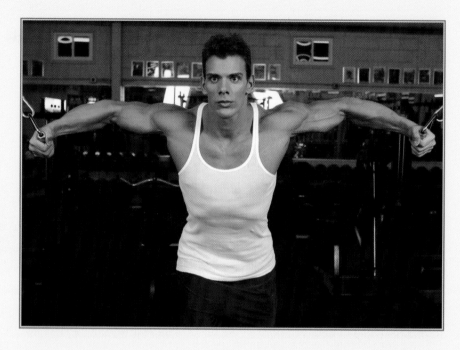

Cable
Crossover

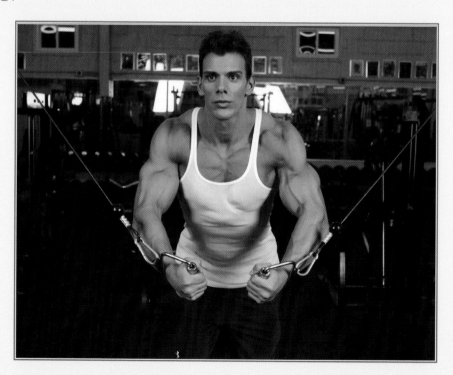

CHEST: SECONDARY EXERCISES

Cable Crossover

(Targets lower-inner/outer pectorals)

This is essentially a standing fly. Attach handles to each of the opposing overhead cables on a twin-cable machine. Grasp the left handle in your left hand and the right handle in your right hand (palms facing up), and stand midway between the two weight stacks with your feet shoulder-width apart. Bend *slightly* forward at your waist to the starting position: elbows bent at 170-degree angles and arms fully extended at your sides. Inhale as you slowly pull the cables together directly in front of you, until the handles meet. Fully contract your pecs for two seconds. Exhale as you slowly let the handles pull your arms back to the starting position.

Perfect form: Keep your head up, with your face straight ahead. Maintain the bend in your elbows (think *bear hug*) as you move the handles through a smooth, controlled arc. Bring the handles far enough back that you're getting a really good stretch.

Advanced tip: I've always gotten the most out of this exercise by really concentrating on the contraction. So make sure that you're squeezing as hard as you can when your hands are together. Concentrate and make every rep equal two.

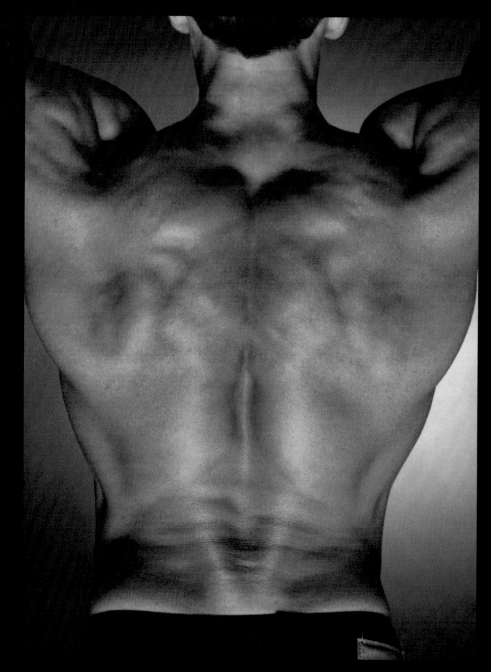

Back

Back

Here's something I hear quite a bit: "Why should I train my back when I can't even see it?"

Well, the back is just as important as any other body part, both in terms of developing a nicely proportioned body and in overall health. In fact, when it comes to performing the basic activities of life, the back is actually more important than most muscle groups.

The back is made up of a number of small to midsize muscles, but for our purposes, we'll simply be focusing on the upper, middle, and lower parts. In my routine, I focus on all three areas: I usually do some sort of pull-down or chin-up to train my upper back, a rowing movement for my middle back, and a hyperextension or dead lift for my lower back. I really focus on bringing my elbows as far back as I can on each movement so that I get a good contraction form every rep.

You must be especially careful to use perfect form when training your back. If you speed up your motion and rely on body momentum to help get out that last rep, you can very easily pull a muscle or even throw your whole back out. If you injure your back, you can't train—at all. So train smart and focus.

I use positive visualization when training my back: I close my eyes and picture my back the way I want it to look. This motivates me to get those last few reps of each set in. I know that if do that, there's a good chance that my back will eventually look like my visualization. Remember, you want to look just as good going as you do coming.

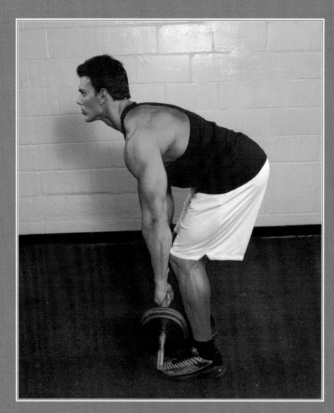

Bent-Over
Row—Barbell

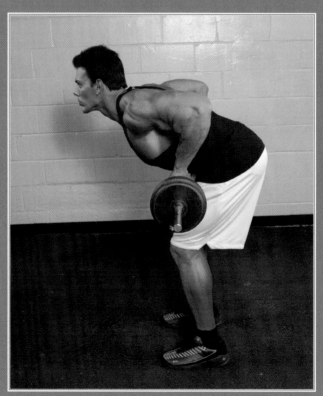

BACK: PRIMARY EXERCISES

Bent-Over Row—Barbell
(Targets upper and lower back)

With a barbell on the floor in front of you, plant your feet shoulder-width apart. Bend over, keeping your back straight and legs slightly bent at the knee, and grasp the bar with your palms facing toward your legs and your hands shoulder-width apart. Keeping your back parallel to the floor, inhale as you slowly lift the bar to your upper abdominals. Slowly lower the bar back to just above the floor as you exhale.

Perfect form: Don't arch your back or bounce up during the exercise. Keep your back straight and parallel to the floor. Hold your head up and face forward, not down.

Variation: Perform the same motion with dumbbells to do the **Bent-over row–dumbbell**: Grasp the dumbbells in an overhand grip with palms facing toward your body, not toward each other.

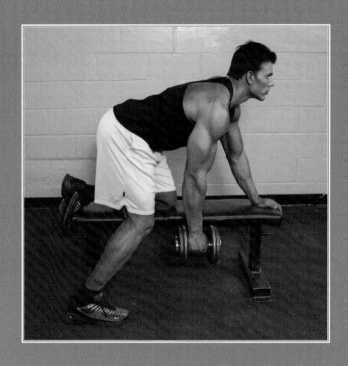

One-Arm
Row—Dumbbell

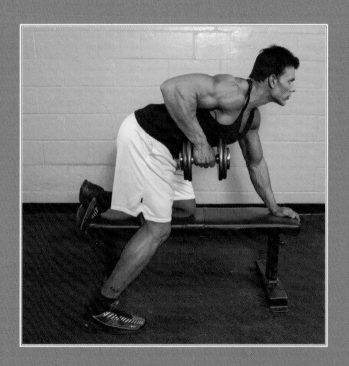

BACK: PRIMARY EXERCISES

One-Arm Row—Dumbbell
(Targets center and lower back)

Stand on the left side of a bench with a dumbbell on the floor in front of you. Rest your right knee and shin on the bench. Bend forward and plant your right hand on the bench, so that your back is parallel to the floor. Grasp the dumbbell with your left hand, palm facing your body. Inhale as you slowly lift the dumbbell up to your side. Exhale as you slowly lower the dumbbell to just above the floor. Finish your reps, move to the right side of the bench, and repeat the exercise with your right arm.

Perfect form: Keep your back straight and parallel to the floor. Face forward, not down, and don't lift your shoulder up. Keep your elbow and the dumbbell in close to your body.

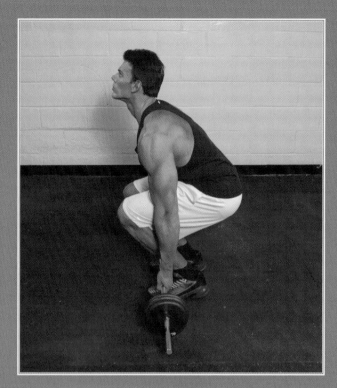

Dead Lift—
Barbell

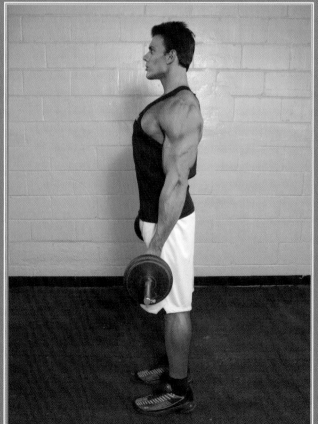

BACK: PRIMARY EXERCISES

Dead Lift—Barbell

(Targets trapezius or "traps," and lower back)

Stand with your knees slightly bent and feet shoulder-width apart, with a barbell in front of you on the floor. Bend over and grasp the bar with one palm toward you and one facing away, hands shoulder-width apart. Keeping your feet flat on the floor, with your shoulders back and your back straight, drop into the starting position: a solid squat with your butt low and pushed back behind you, your knees over your feet and your thighs parallel to the floor. Inhale as you stand back up, lifting the bar to your upper thigh by driving the weight up from your heels through your thighs and butt (sitting back will help you do this). Exhale as you slowly drop back into your squat, lowering the bar toward the floor.

Perfect form: As you squat, keep your butt low to the ground—don't shoot it up in the air. Rounding your back can lead to serious injury. Push from your heels, not the balls of your feet.

Advanced tip: This is a power move, one of the rare exercises where your motion shouldn't be uniformly slow. Descend slowly, but once you've practiced the motion and have developed good form, you should press up from the ground explosively.

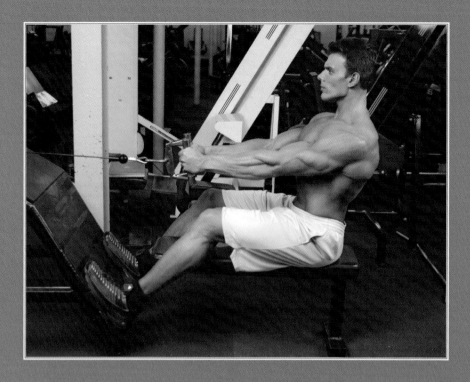

Row—Cable
with V-Handle

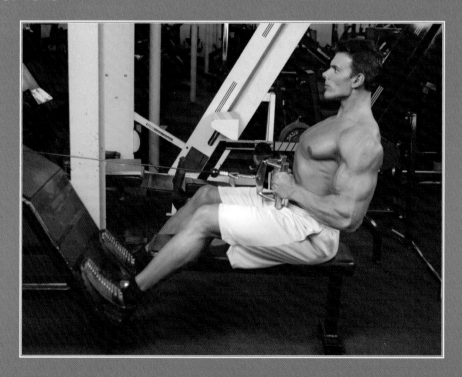

BACK: PRIMARY EXERCISES

Row—Cable with V-Handle

(Targets center and lower latissimus dorsi, or "lats")

Attach a V-handle to a low cable. Sit on the bench with your feet braced against the foot-pads shoulder-width apart. Bend your knees, lean forward, and grasp both sides of the handle. Pushing against the footpads, slide your butt back until your knees are just slightly bent, and lean back until your torso is vertical. Without moving your torso, inhale as you slowly pull the handle back into your abs. Exhale and slowly allow the handle to move back toward the weight stack until your arms are fully extended.

Perfect form: Once you've pushed back to the starting position, don't move your legs or shift your torso from vertical. Keep your chest high and your shoulders pulled back throughout the motion, but don't lean your torso forward or back.

Variation: For a wider grip, instead of the V-handle, attach a bar to the cable to do a **Row—cable with bar**.

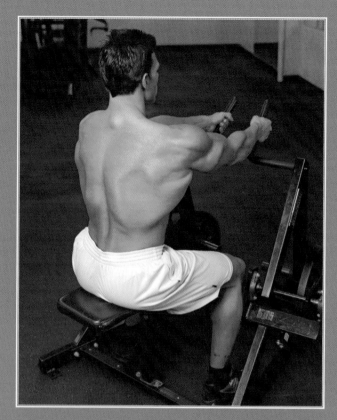

Row—
Machine

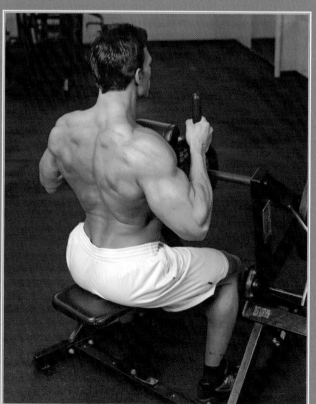

BACK: PRIMARY EXERCISES

Row—Machine
(Targets lower or upper lats)

(Machines will vary.) Sit on the bench, your torso tight against the chest pad. Grasp the handles and slowly pull them back to your sides as you inhale. Slowly return the handles to the starting position as you exhale.

Perfect form: Pull your shoulders back, but keep your chest firmly against the chest pad throughout the exercise.

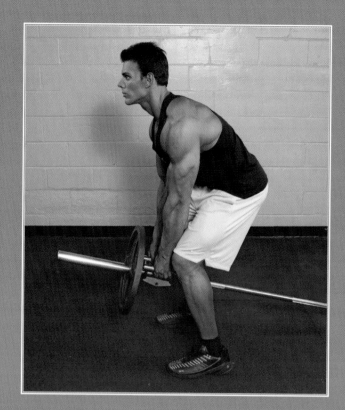

Row—T-Bar

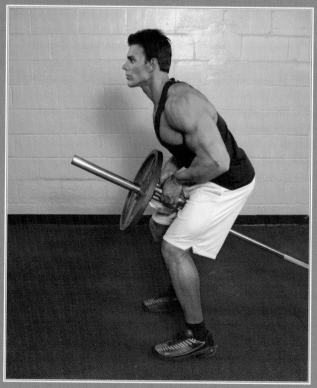

Row—T-Bar

(Targets middle and outer back)

Plant your feet shoulder-width apart on the foot board, keeping your knees slightly bent. Grasp the handles of the T-bar and slowly pull them back to your sides as you inhale. Slowly return the handles to the starting position as you exhale.

Perfect form: Pull your shoulders back throughout the exercise.

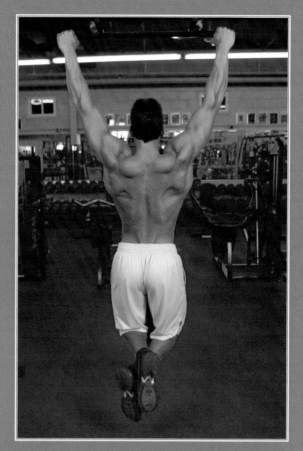

Chin-Up

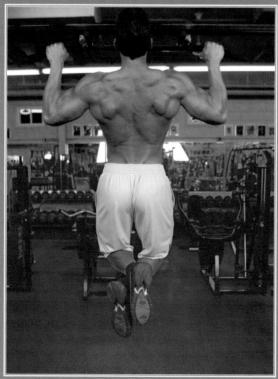

BACK: PRIMARY EXERCISES

Chin-Up

(Targets upper and outer back)

Grasp a chin bar (either a straight bar or one with the handles angled downward) with palms facing away from you and hands shoulder-width apart. Bend your knees and lift your feet behind you, so that your body is hanging from the bar. As you inhale, slowly pull your body up until your chin is above the bar. Exhale as you lower your body back down until your arms are fully extended.

Perfect form: Perform the exercise slowly, without jerking your body up or bouncing up from the bottom position. Don't swing your body to gain momentum—keep it hanging straight down.

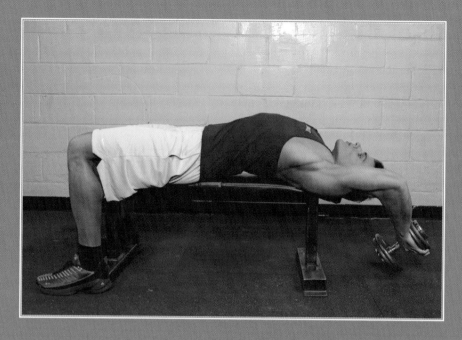

Dumbbell
Pullover

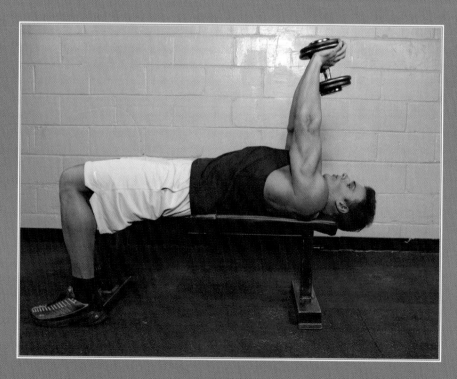

BACK: PRIMARY EXERCISES

Dumbbell Pullover
(Targets lower lats)

Stand a dumbbell on its end at the foot of a flat bench. Lay your shoulders and upper back on the bench, with your head hanging over one side and your feet comfortably planted shoulder-width apart on the other side. Reach over and grasp the top of the dumbbell from below so that the grip is sandwiched between both thumbs and forefingers and your palms are flat against the plates. Lift the dumbbell onto your chest. Inhale as you lift the dumbbell off your chest until your arms are fully extended (but elbows aren't locked), then slowly lower the dumbbell behind your head, keeping your arms almost straight. Exhale as you lift the dumbbell back up above your chest.

Perfect form: Keep your arms straight throughout the exercise, and don't arch your back. Keep your knees bent and your hips lower than the bench.

Variation: **Pullover machine.**

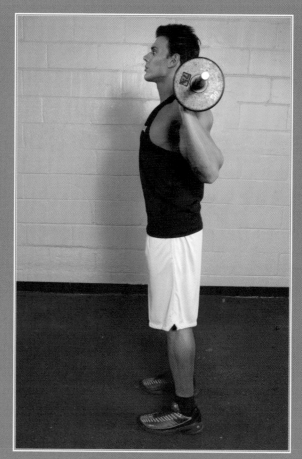

Good Morning
—Barbell

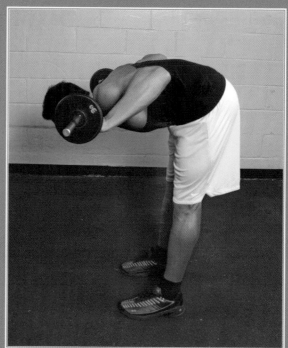

BACK: SECONDARY EXERCISES

Good Morning—Barbell
(Targets lower back, spinal erectors)

Place a barbell behind your neck, resting across your shoulders. Extend your arms straight out to your sides and hang your hands over the ends of the barbell. Stand with your feet shoulder-width apart, and inhale as you bend at your hips and slowly lower your torso until it's parallel to the floor. Exhale as you slowly lift your upper body back to the starting position.

Perfect form: It's easy to injure your lower back with poor form, so keep your knees and back straight. Go slow; don't jerk the weight up. Use light to moderate weight.

Advanced tips: Don't lean forward past horizontal—you might not be able to get back up. And keep your motion fluid.

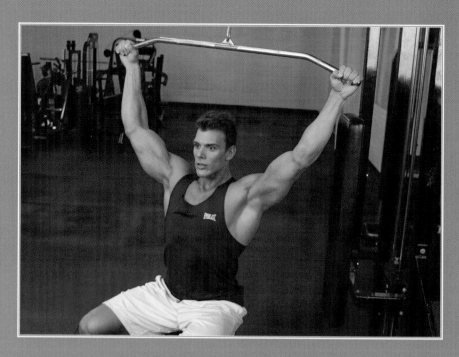

Lat Pull-Down—
Front

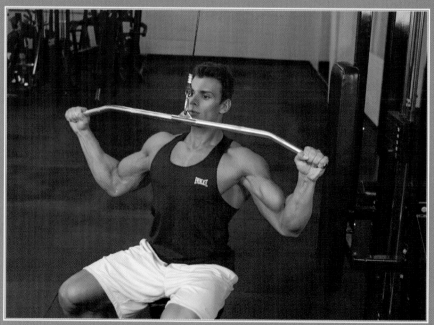

BACK: SECONDARY EXERCISES

Lat Pull-Down—Front
(Targets lats)

Attach a straight bar to an overhead cable. Grasp the bar with hands shoulder-width apart and palms facing away from you. Extend your arms fully as you sit down facing the machine, and lock your thighs under the thigh pads. Facing forward with your chest up, pinch your shoulder blades together and inhale as you slowly pull the bar down in front of you to just below your chin. Exhale as you slowly return the bar to the starting position, fully extending your arms to stretch out your lats.

Perfect form: Keep a slight arch in your back so you can pull your elbows slightly back on way down, but don't lean back. And *definitely* don't rock your torso back and forth—use a slow, controlled motion. Don't pull down much past your chin because that moves the work to your biceps.

Advanced tip: Pretend that you don't have hands and are pulling with your elbows. I get a much better contraction when I do this.

Variations: The **Reverse-grip lat pull-down** uses an almost identical motion and form, but you grasp the bar with an underhand grip and can bring the bar down to your upper chest. Follow the same good-form tips as above, plus keep your elbows tucked in close to your sides. Experienced bodybuilders often perform a **Rear lat pull-down**, bringing the bar down behind their heads. It's a classic exercise but places more strain on the shoulder joint, which can lead to rotator-cuff injuries. Pay close attention to your form, and use a very controlled motion if you try this variation.

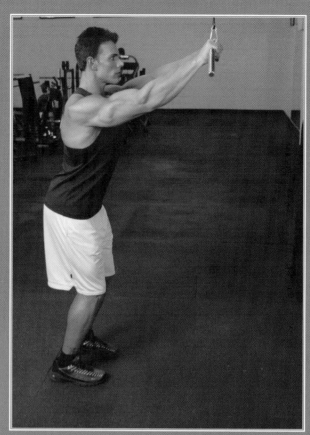

Stiff-Arm Lat
Pull-Down

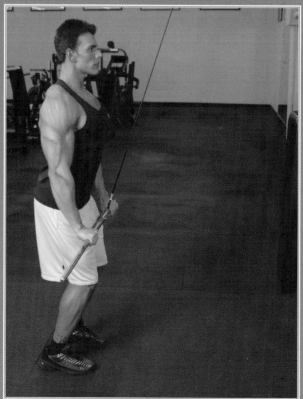

BACK: SECONDARY EXERCISES

Stiff-Arm Lat Pull-Down
(Targets upper back)

Attach a wide-grip bar to an overhead cable. Stand facing the machine, with shoulders back and feet shoulder-width apart. Grasp the bar with hands wider than shoulder-width apart and palms facing away from you. Keeping your arms straight (without locking your elbows), inhale as you slowly push the bar down toward your thighs. Exhale as you slowly return the bar to the starting position.

Perfect form: Keep your arms straight so that you don't bring your shoulders, chest, and arms into play. Move slowly, and don't hunch forward. Control the bar—don't let it control you.

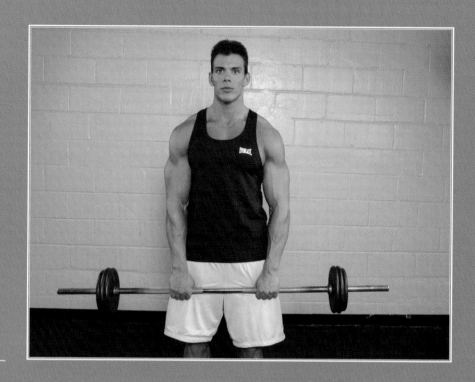

Shrug—
Barbell

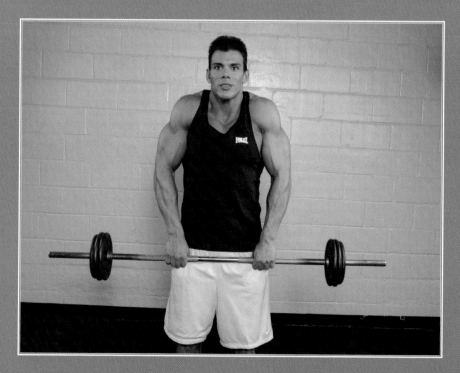

BACK: SECONDARY EXERCISES

Shrug–Barbell
(Targets traps)

Grasp a barbell in an overhand grip with hands shoulder-width apart. With feet shoulder-width apart and arms fully extended downward, hold the bar in front of you. Inhale as you slowly lift your shoulders as high as possible (making an exaggerated shrugging motion), lifting the bar. Don't move anything but your shoulders. Exhale as you slowly lower your shoulders and the bar back to the starting position.

Perfect form: Lift only with your shoulders, not your arms. Keep your back as straight as you can, and don't rock backward as you lift.

Advanced tip: Pause at the top and bottom of the motion for a second to intensify the burn.

Variations: Use the same motion and form for the **Shrug–dumbbell** exercise; just substitute two dumbbells for the barbell. You can also perform a **Seated shrug–dumbbell** to help restrict the motion to your shoulders.

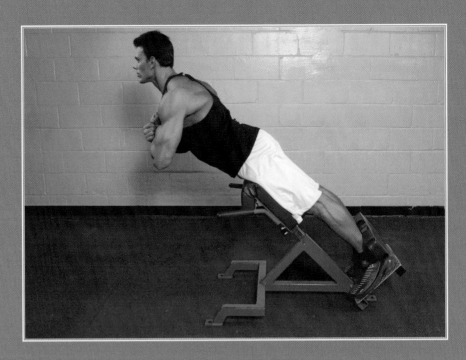

Hyperextension—
Machine

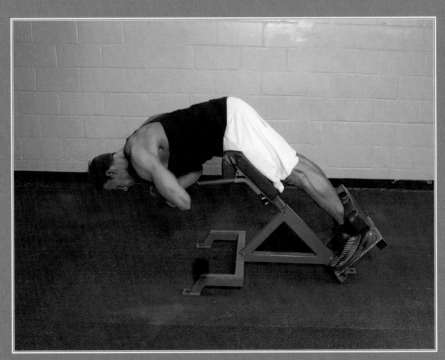

BACK: SECONDARY EXERCISES

Hyperextension—Machine
(Targets lower back, spinal erectors)

Lean your pelvis against the pad and place your feet on the footplate, with your heels against the heel pad and your toes pointed forward. Fold your hands across your chest and lean forward. Inhale as you slowly lower your torso forward, bending until your hips form a 60-degree angle. Exhale as you slowly lift your torso back to the starting position.

Perfect form: Make sure that you lock your lower body into place. It should be immobile. Move slowly—don't bounce up and down.

Advanced tip: Hold a weight in your arms to increase the intensity of this exercise.

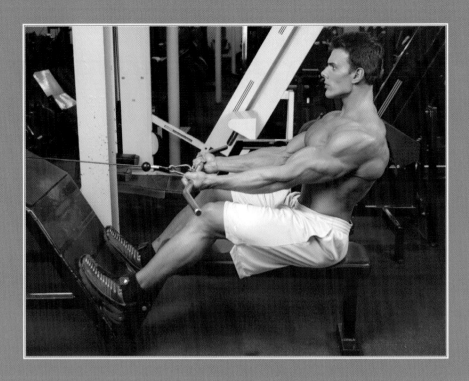

Reverse-Grip Row—
Cable with Straight Bar

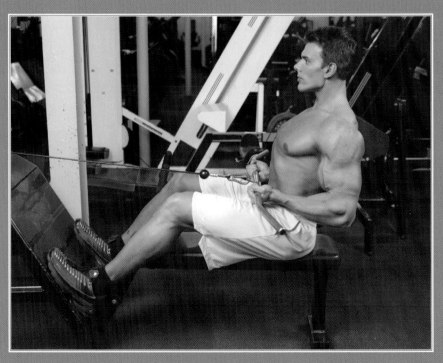

Front Military Press—Barbell

(Targets entire shoulder)

Sit with your feet flat on the floor and your back firmly against the backrest. Grasp the bar with palms facing forward, hands shoulder-width apart. Lift the bar off its rests and over your head. Inhale as you slowly lower the bar in front of your face until your hands are just above shoulder height. Exhale as you slowly press the bar back up over your head until your arms are fully extended (but elbows aren't locked).

Perfect form: Keep your back flat against the rest throughout the exercise. Don't bounce the bar up from its lowest position.

Variations: For extra safety, especially when you don't have a spotter, you can use the same motion and form on a Smith machine to do a **Front military press–Smith machine** exercise. Either exercise can also be performed standing.

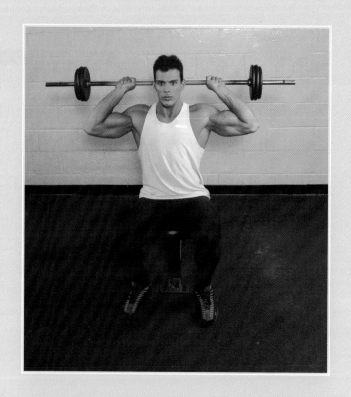

Rear Military
Press—
Barbell

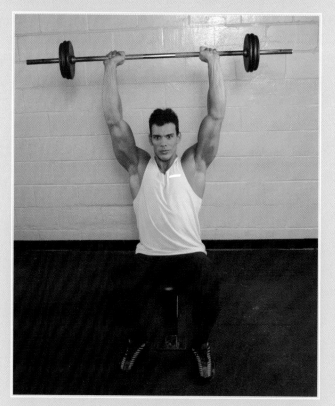

Rear Military Press—Barbell

(Targets entire shoulder)

Sit with your feet flat on the floor, your back firmly against the backrest. Grasp the bar with palms facing forward, hands shoulder-width apart. Lift the bar off its rests and over your head. Inhale as you slowly lower the bar behind your head until it's even with the bottom of your ears. Exhale as you slowly press the bar back up over your head until your arms are fully extended (but elbows aren't locked).

Perfect form: Keep your back flat against the rest throughout the exercise. Don't bounce the bar up from its lowest position.

Variations: For extra safety, especially when you don't have a spotter, you can use the same motion and form on a Smith machine to do a **Rear military press–Smith machine**. With either, the exercise can also be performed standing.

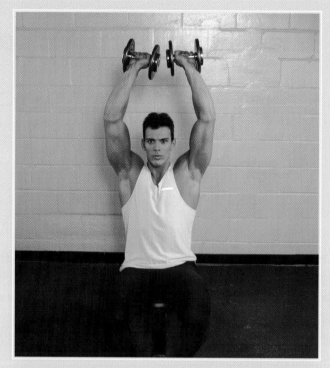

Shoulder Press—
Dumbbell

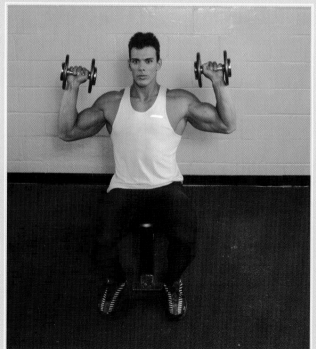

SHOULDERS: PRIMARY EXERCISES

Shoulder Press—Dumbbell
(Targets entire shoulder)

Sit with your feet flat on the floor and a dumbbell in each hand, resting upright on your thighs. Lift the dumbbells up to just above your shoulders, rotating them so that they're parallel to the floor, your palms facing forward and your elbows directly below your wrists. Inhale as you slowly press the barbells up until your arms are fully extended (but elbows aren't locked). Then exhale as you slowly lower the dumbbells back to just above your shoulders.

Perfect form: Keep your back flat against the bench throughout the exercise. Don't bounce the dumbbells up from their lowest position.

Shoulder Press—Machine (Variation)
(Targets entire shoulder)

Adjust the seat so that the machine's handles are just above shoulder height. Sit with your feet flat on the floor and your back firmly against the backrest. Grasp the handles, and inhale as you slowly press the handles up until your arms are fully extended (but elbows aren't locked). Exhale as you slowly lower the handles back to just above shoulder height.

Perfect form: Keep your back flat against the back pad throughout the exercise. Don't bounce the handles up from their lowest position.

Advanced tip: Some machines have only one set of grips, others have both a pair of grips that you grasp with palms facing forward and a pair of parallel grips that you grasp with palms facing each other. Use the parallel grips to place less stress on the shoulder joints.

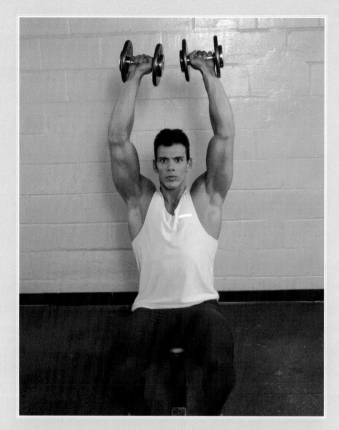

Arnold
Press—
Dumbbell

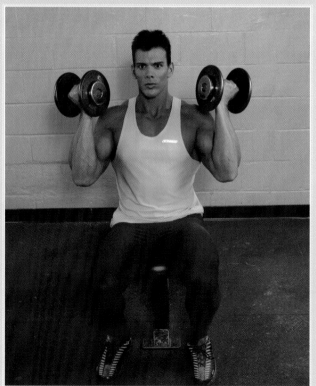

Arnold Press—Dumbbell

(Targets entire shoulder)

Sit with your feet flat on the floor and a dumbbell in each hand, resting upright on your thighs. Lift the dumbbells up to just above your shoulders, rotating them so that they're parallel to the floor, your palms facing back toward you and your elbows directly below your wrists. Inhale as you slowly press the dumbbells up until your arms are fully extended (but elbows aren't locked). As you press the dumbbells up, rotate them so that at full arm extension your palms are facing forward. Exhale as you slowly lower the dumbbells back to just above your shoulders, rotating them so that your palms again face toward you.

Perfect form: Keep your back flat against the bench throughout the exercise. Don't bounce the dumbbells up from their lowest position.

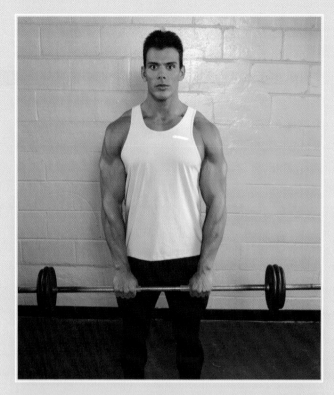

Upright Row—
Barbell

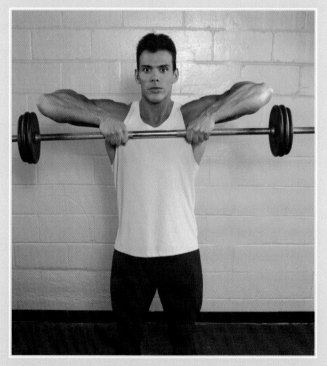

SHOULDERS: PRIMARY EXERCISES

Upright Row—Barbell
(Targets side deltoids or "delts")

Stand with feet shoulder-width apart and knees slightly bent, a barbell in front of you. Bend over and grasp the bar with an overhand grip and hands about 6–8 inches apart. Lifting from your legs to avoid back strain, stand back upright to the starting position so that the bar rests across your upper thighs. Inhale as you slowly lift the bar up to your chin, your elbows pushing straight out to your sides, your hands keeping the bar as close to your body as possible throughout the lift. Exhale as you slowly lower the bar to your upper thighs, again keeping it right next to your body.

Perfect form: Keep your back straight and your head up. Don't lift the bar forward, away from your body; don't bounce the bar up from its lowest position; and don't rock your shoulders back as you lift. Move only your arms.

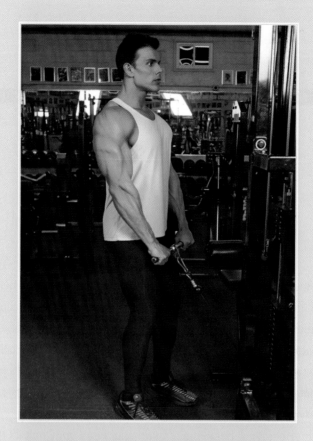

Upright
Row—Cable

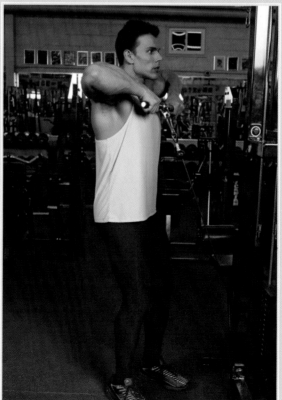

SHOULDERS: PRIMARY EXERCISES

Upright Row—Cable
(Targets side delts)

Attach a straight bar to a lower cable. Stand with your feet shoulder-width apart and knees slightly bent, as close to the pulley as possible. Bend over and grasp the bar with your palms facing toward you and your hands about 6–8 inches apart. Lifting from your legs to avoid back strain, stand back upright to the starting position so that the bar rests across your upper thighs. Inhale as you slowly lift the bar up to your chin, your elbows pushing straight out to your sides, your hands keeping the bar as close to your body as possible throughout the lift. Exhale as you slowly lower the bar to your upper thighs, again keeping it right next to your body.

Perfect form: Keep your back straight and your head up. Don't lift the bar forward, away from your body; don't bounce the bar up from its lowest position; and don't rock your shoulders back as you lift. Move only your arms.

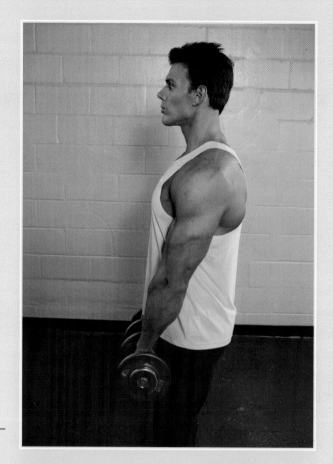

Front Raise— Dumbbell

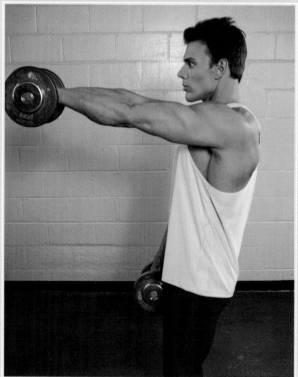

SHOULDERS: SECONDARY EXERCISES

Front Raise–Dumbbell

(Targets front delts)

Grasp dumbbells in both hands. Stand with your shoulders back, back straight, knees slightly bent, and feet shoulder-width apart. Hold the dumbbells in front of your thighs with your arms fully extended (elbows slightly bent) and your palms facing your legs. With your elbow fixed in a 10- to 30-degree angle, inhale as you lift your left arm until the dumbbell is at eye level. Exhale as you slowly lower the dumbbell to the starting position, and then repeat the exercise with your right arm. Alternate arms until your set is complete.

Perfect form: Keep your knees slightly bent to take pressure off your lower back, but don't bounce from your legs as you lift. Move only your arms, and maintain the bend in your elbows. Don't lift the dumbbell higher than eye level.

Advanced tip: For a killer pump, hold each dumbbell at eye level for two seconds at the top of the motion.

Variations: To work both shoulders at once, try the **Front raise–barbell**: Follow the same form and motion, but substitute a light barbell for the dumbbells. For perfectly consistent resistance throughout the exercise, try the **Front raise–cable**: Use the same motion and form to lift a handle attached to a lower cable as you face away from the machine. You'll have to do one arm at a time—you won't be able to alternate—but that will only intensify the burn.

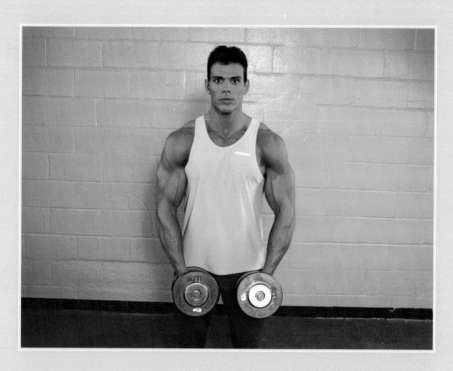

Side Raise—
Dumbbell

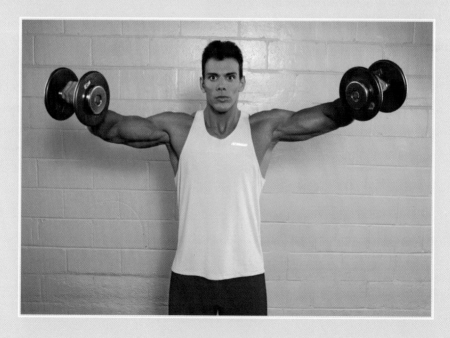

Side Raise–Dumbbell

(Targets side delts)

Hold two dumbbells next to your thighs with your arms fully extended. Have a slight bend in your elbows and your palms facing each other. Standing with your knees slightly bent and your feet shoulder-width apart, bend very slightly forward at the hips. Inhale as you slowly lift both dumbbells directly out to your sides until your elbows are at shoulder height. Your palms should be facing down. Exhale as you slowly lower the dumbbells back to your sides.

Perfect form: Keep your knees slightly bent to take pressure off your lower back, but don't bounce from your legs as you lift. Move only your arms, and maintain the bend in your elbows. Don't lift the dumbbell higher than your shoulders.

Advanced tip: For a killer pump, hold each dumbbell at shoulder level for two seconds at the top of the motion.

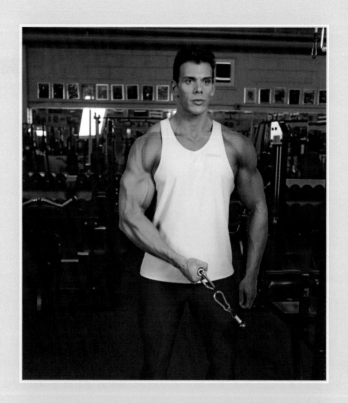

Side Raise—
Cable

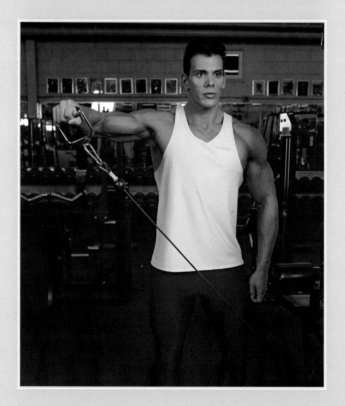

SHOULDERS: SECONDARY EXERCISES

Side Raise—Cable

(Targets side delts)

Attach a stirrup handle to a low cable. Stand perpendicular to the machine with your right side facing the weight stack. Bend over and grasp the stirrup in your left hand with your palm facing up. Stand up so that your knees are slightly bent and your feet are shoulder-width apart, pulling the cable into the starting position. Your left arm should be fully extended (elbow slightly bent) and down in front of your thighs. Brace yourself against the machine with your right arm. Inhale as you slowly lift the stirrup straight out to your left side and until your elbow is at shoulder level. Exhale as you slowly lower the stirrup to the starting position. Finish your reps and perform the exercise with your right arm.

Perfect form: Keep your knees slightly bent to take pressure off your lower back, but don't bounce from your legs as you lift. Move only your arm, and maintain the bend in your elbow. Don't lift the stirrup higher than your shoulder.

Advanced tips: For a killer pump, hold each cable at shoulder level for two seconds at the top of the motion. This exercise can be performed either with the cable in front of your body or behind it. I like to alternate front and back from workout to workout to keep the exercise fresh and to help prevent myself from cheating.

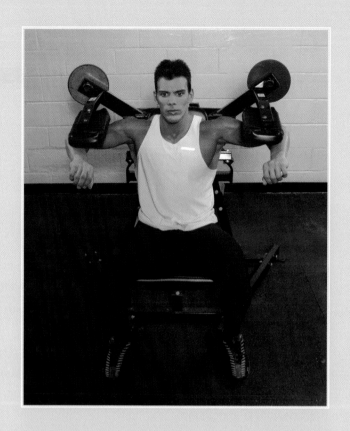

Side Raise Machine

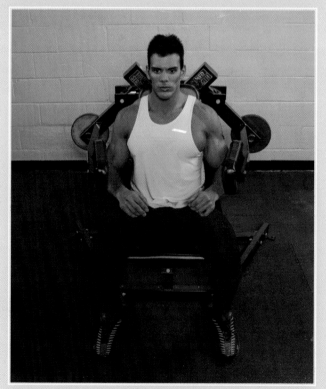

SHOULDERS: SECONDARY EXERCISES

Side Raise—Machine

(Targets side delts)

Sit with your back firmly against the backrest and your elbows under the arm pads. Inhale as you slowly lift the arm pads up to shoulder level. Exhale as you slowly lower the pads to the starting position.

Perfect form: Look forward and keep your back straight. Don't lift the pads higher than your shoulders or you'll be shifting the stress from your delts to your traps. If you're using a machine where you face in, keep your chest flat against the chest pad.

Advanced tip: Again, holding for two seconds at the top of the motion will intensify your burn.

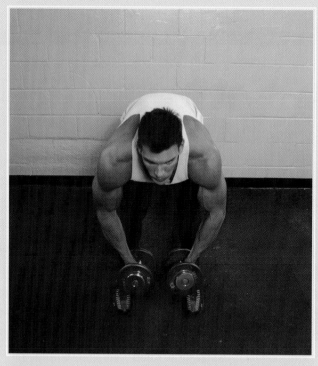

Standing Bent-Over
Raise—Dumbbell

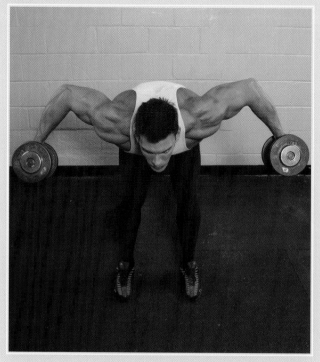

SHOULDERS: SECONDARY EXERCISES

Standing Bent-Over Raise—Dumbbell

(Targets rear delts)

Stand with your feet shoulder-width apart, knees slightly bent. Holding a dumbbell in each hand, bend forward at the waist to the starting position: torso parallel to the floor, palms facing each other, and elbows bent at an 150-degree angle. Maintaining that elbow position (think *bear hug*), inhale as you lift your arms until your elbows are at shoulder height. Exhale as you return the dumbbells to the starting position.

Perfect form: Don't rock up and down. Keep your torso horizontal, and move only your arms to keep from cheating with your biceps. Keep your elbows fixed at their 150-degree angle and concentrate on lifting from the elbows.

Advanced tip: Pull your elbows back as far as possible at the top of the motion, and then squeeze your rear delts hard as you can.

Variation: For consistent resistance throughout the entire exercise, try the **Bent-over raise–cable**: Attach handles to opposing lower cables on a twin-cable machine. Grasp the handle on your left with your right hand, palm facing up, and grasp the right handle, palm up with your left hand. Stand midway between the two cables, bend forward at the waist, and duplicate the motion and form above.

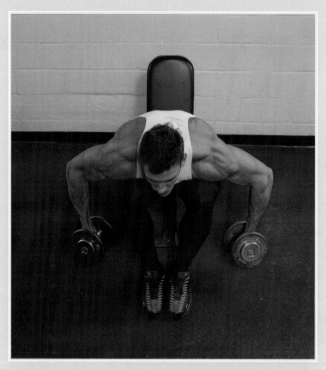

Seated Bent-Over
Raise—Dumbbell

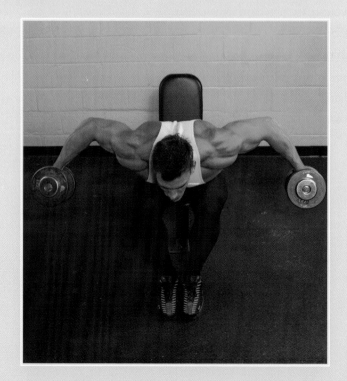

SHOULDERS: SECONDARY EXERCISES

Seated Bent-Over Raise–Dumbbell

(Targets rear delts)

Sit on the end of a bench with two dumbbells on the floor at your sides. Plant your feet flat on the floor, close together and beyond your knees. Lean forward to the starting position, resting your torso on your thighs. With palms facing each other, grasp a dumbbell in each hand under your thighs. Your elbows should be fixed at 150-degree angles (think *bear hug*). Maintaining that bend in your elbows, inhale as you slowly lift your arms out to your sides, perpendicular to your torso, until the dumbbells are at shoulder height. Exhale as you slowly lower the dumbbells back to the starting position.

Perfect form: Don't bounce up and down. Keep your torso flat against your thighs, and move only your arms to keep from cheating with your biceps. Keep your elbows fixed at their 150-degree angles, and concentrate on lifting from the elbows.

Advanced tip: Pull your elbows back as far as possible at the top of the motion, and then squeeze your rear delts hard as you can.

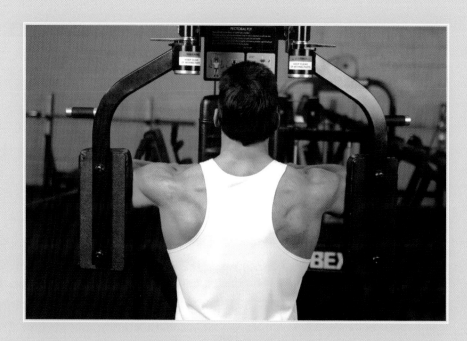

Reverse Fly—
Pec Deck

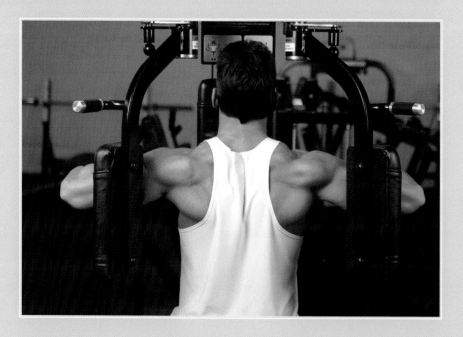

SHOULDERS: SECONDARY EXERCISES

Reverse Fly–Pec Deck

(Targets rear delts)

(Machines will vary.) Sit facing the pad, with your chest firmly against it. Grasp the handles with your thumbs at the top of your hands and your arms parallel to the floor. Fix your elbows at 150-degree angles (think *bear hug*). Maintaining that bend in your elbows, inhale as you slowly pull the handles back as far as you can. Exhale as you slowly return the handles to the starting position.

Perfect form: Keep your chest up against the pad and your elbows fixed in a bent position throughout the exercise.

Advanced tip: When you've got your elbows pulled all the way back, hold the position for a second or two and squeeze your rear delts as hard as you can.

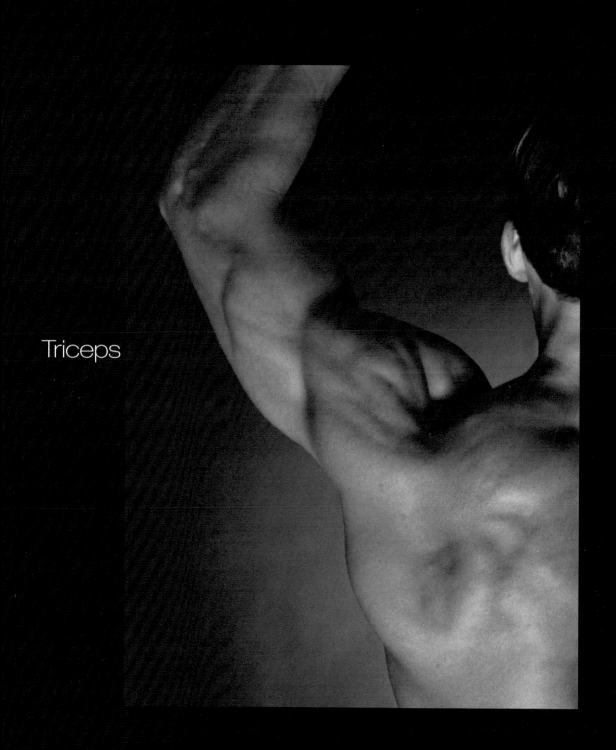

Triceps

Triceps

Just like Rodney Dangerfield, this part of the body gets "no respect." When people think of powerful arms, most of them don't think of triceps—instead, they focus on biceps. Why? Because the biceps are in the front and because it's what we show off when someone tells us to "make a muscle." For these reasons, many people who are new to weight training might feel that there's no real urgency to developing their triceps. Well, I strongly urge *you* to take your triceps training seriously.

Triceps exercises are all very targeted. Just like with biceps, the most important thing to do is to concentrate on using only the muscle itself—don't cheat with your shoulder, back, or chest. You have to do these exercises with perfect form or you won't benefit from them in any way. Fortunately, you have a secret weapon when training your triceps: These exercises are the only ones that break the "no lock-out rule"—that is, when you train the triceps, not only should you lock out your elbow for a moment at the peak of the motion, it's absolutely necessary if you want to get a full contraction.

As long as you keep your motion slow and controlled, locking out on triceps exercises isn't dangerous. You won't injure your elbow. So lock out those elbows, get a full contraction, and be amazed by the definition you get on the upper part of your arms.

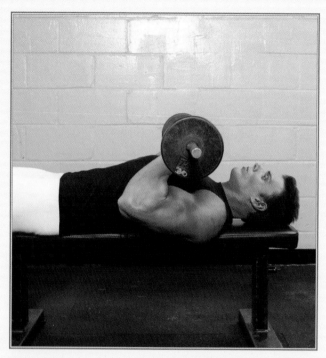

Narrow-Grip Bench
Press—Barbell

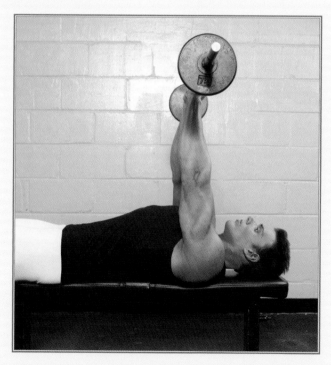

TRICEPS: PRIMARY EXERCISES

Narrow-Grip Bench Press—Barbell

(Targets overall triceps)

Lie on a bench with your feet flat on the ground. Grasp the bar in an overhand grip with hands 6–8 inches apart. Exhaling, lift the bar off its rests and slowly lower it to mid-chest. Without resting the bar on your chest or bouncing the bar up off of it, inhale as you slowly press the bar up until your arms are fully extended.

Perfect form: Keep your back flat on the bench throughout the exercise—don't arch upward.

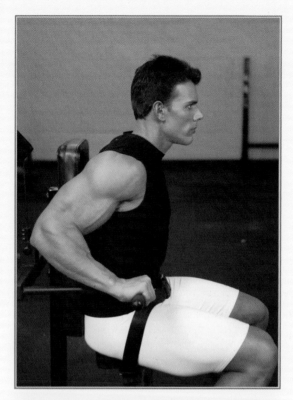

Triceps Dip—
Machine

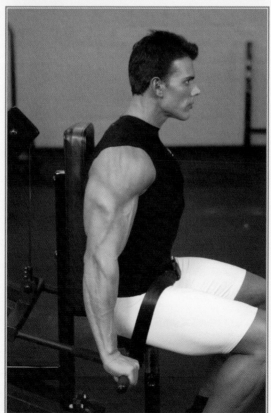

TRICEPS: PRIMARY EXERCISES

Triceps Dip—Machine

(Targets overall triceps)

Adjust the seat so that the handles are about even with the bottom of your chest. Be sure you can grasp the handles at your sides when you're sitting down flat. Sit down and grasp the handles. Inhale as you slowly press the handles down until your arms are fully extended. Exhale as you slowly let the handles return to the starting position.

Perfect form: Keep your body weight firmly on the seat and your back against the back pad throughout—and if the machine has a seat belt, use it.

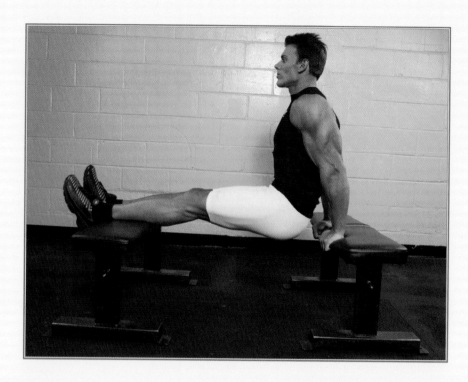

Triceps Dip—
Two Benches

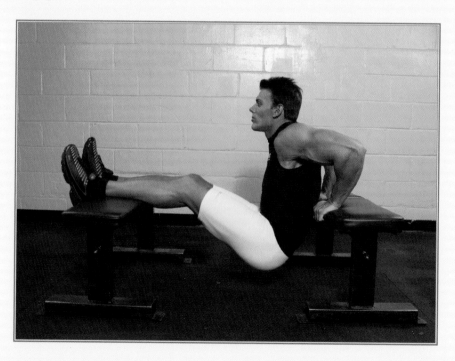

TRICEPS: PRIMARY EXERCISES

Triceps Dip—Two Benches

(Targets area near elbow)

Place two benches parallel to each other at a distance a little shorter than the length of your legs. Sit on the edge of one bench facing the other. With both hands, grasp the bench you're sitting on. Place your hands close to your butt, lean your weight back onto your arms, and shift your butt forward and off the bench as you lift your heels onto the other bench. Inhale as you slowly lower your torso by your arms until your elbows are almost even with your shoulders. Exhale as you slowly lift your torso back up until your arms are fully extended and your elbows lock.

Perfect form: Go as low as you can, and push all the way back up until your elbows are locked—then hold the position and contract your triceps for a second.

Advanced tip: You can increase the difficulty of your dips by having a partner place weight plates on your thighs once your feet are up on the second bench.

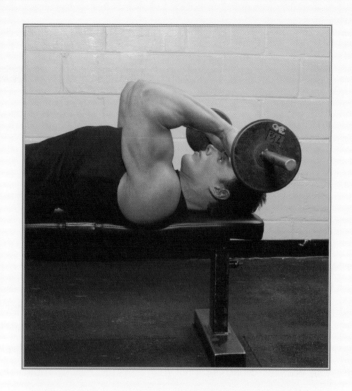

Skullcrushers—
Barbell

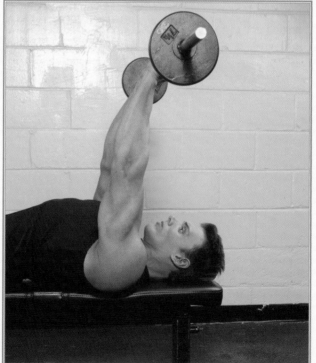

TRICEPS: PRIMARY EXERCISES

Skullcrushers—Barbell
(Targets overall triceps)

Balance a bar on the very end of a flat bench. Lie on your back on the bench with your feet flat on the floor and your head almost touching the bar. Raise your hands above your head, elbows pointing up, and grasp the bar with your palms facing up, shoulder-width apart. Without moving your biceps, inhale and slowly lift the bar up until your elbows are locked. Then exhale as you slowly lower the bar back down and below the bench, as far as you comfortably can without moving your upper arms.

Perfect form: Keep your biceps immobile, with your elbows in tight and not pointing out away from your sides.

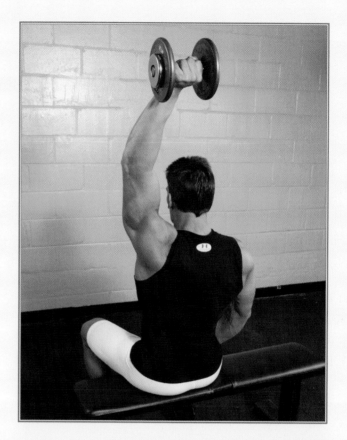

Overhead
Triceps
Extension—
Dumbbell

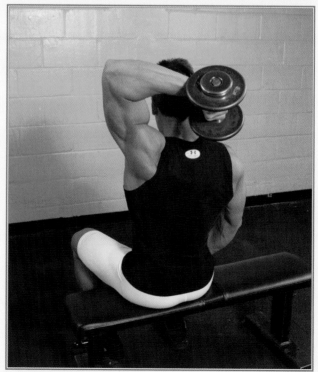

TRICEPS: PRIMARY EXERCISES

Overhead Triceps Extension– Dumbbell
(Targets overall triceps)

Stand with feet shoulder-width apart and knees slightly bent, with a dumbbell in your left hand and your right arm at your side. Raise the dumbbell so that your left arm is extended straight up. Keeping your upper arm pointed straight up, inhale as you slowly lower the dumbbell back behind your head. Then exhale as you lift the dumbbell back up until your arm is fully extended, your elbow locked. Complete your reps, switch arms, and perform the exercise with your right arm.

Perfect form: The key to this extension is keeping your biceps immobile with your elbow pointing straight up. Move *only* your triceps.

Variations: You can exercise both arms simultaneously with two dumbbells, if you watch your form carefully. To eliminate unnecessary upper-body motion and better isolate the triceps, try the **Seated overhead triceps extension–dumbbell**: Just use the same motion and form while seated on a bench with a short backrest.

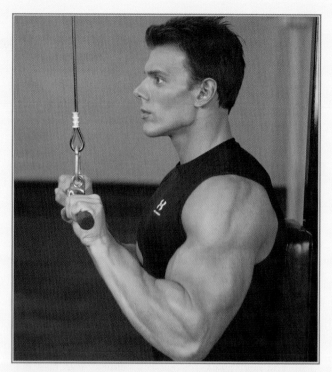

Two-Arm Cable Push-Down— Straight Bar

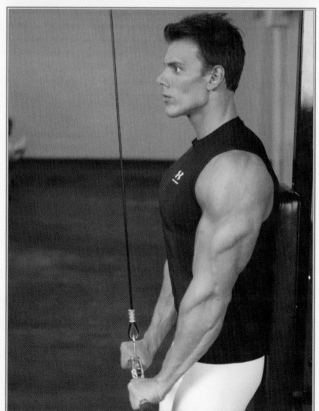

TRICEPS: PRIMARY EXERCISES

Two-Arm Cable Push-Down— Straight Bar
(Targets overall triceps)

Attach a straight bar to a high cable. Stand with feet shoulder-width apart and knees slightly bent. If the cable station has a backrest, use it. Grasp the bar with palms facing down and hands shoulder-width apart. Pull the bar down to the starting position: upper arms straight down at your sides and forearms straight out in front of you, parallel to the floor. Inhale as you slowly push the bar down toward your thighs until your arms are fully extended, your elbows locked out. Move only your forearms. Exhale as you slowly allow the bar to rise back up to the starting position.

Perfect form: Keep your back straight—don't hunch over to cheat with your shoulders and chest as you push down. Keep your elbows at your side and pointing straight down.

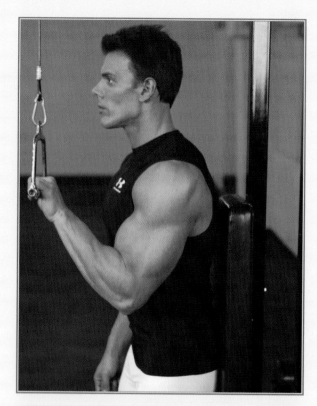

One-Arm
Cable
Push-Down

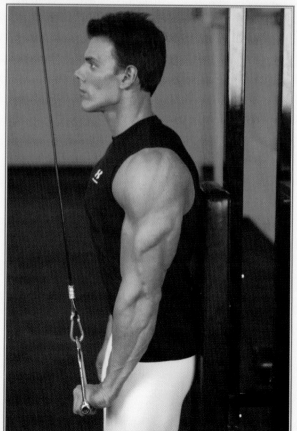

TRICEPS: PRIMARY EXERCISES

One-Arm Cable Push-Down

(Targets overall triceps)

Attach a handle to a high cable. Stand with feet shoulder-width apart and knees slightly bent. If the cable station has a backrest, use it. Grasp the handle with your left hand, palm facing down. Pull the handle down to the starting position: upper arm at your side and forearm straight out in front of you, parallel to the floor. Inhale as you slowly push the handle down toward your thigh until your arm is fully extended and your elbow locks. Move only your forearm. Exhale as you slowly allow the handle to rise back up to the starting position. Complete your reps, switch arms, and repeat the exercise with your right arm.

Perfect form: Keep your back straight—don't hunch over to cheat with your shoulders and chest as you push down. Keep your elbow at your side, pointing straight down.

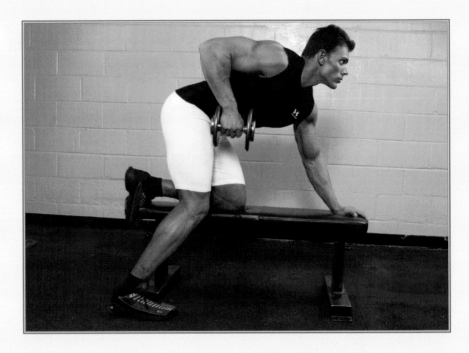

Kickback—
Dumbbell

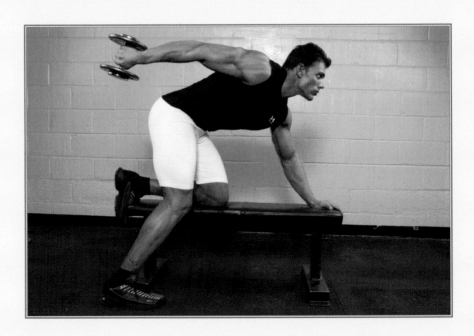

TRICEPS: SECONDARY EXERCISES

Kickback—Dumbbell
(Targets triceps brachii)

Stand on the left side of a flat bench with a dumbbell on the floor in front of you. Rest your right knee and shin on the bench. Bend forward and plant your right hand on the bench so that your back is parallel to the floor. Grasp the dumbbell with your left hand, palm facing your body, and lift it to the starting position: upper arm parallel to the floor and elbow tucked into your side. Inhale as you slowly extend your arm until it's pointing straight behind you. Exhale as you slowly lower the dumbbell to the starting position. Finish your reps, move to the right side of the bench, and repeat the exercise with your right arm.

Perfect form: Momentum is your enemy here. Don't swing your arm up and down—instead, use a slow, controlled motion. Keep your elbow locked into position during the movement so that your upper arm stays parallel to the floor. Think of your arm as a hinge. Keep your back straight and parallel to the floor. Face forward, not down.

Advanced tip: You don't need a lot of weight here. Focus on form. The farther you can kick the dumbbell out—the closer you get to full extension of your arm—the better the contraction.

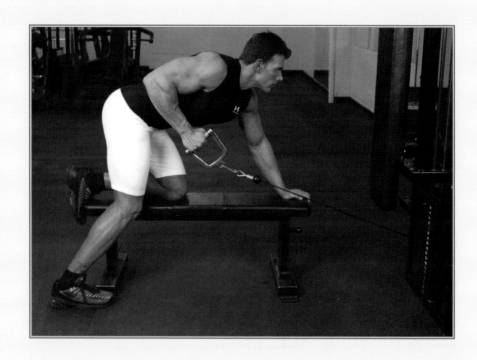

Kickback—
Cable

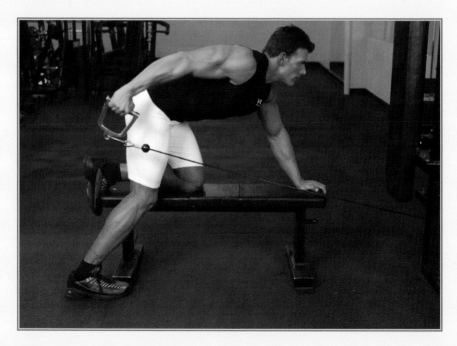

TRICEPS: SECONDARY EXERCISES

Kickback–Cable

(Targets overall triceps)

Attach a handle to a low cable. Position a bench in front of the machine, perpendicular to it and far enough to the right side of the pulley that the cable can be pulled out next to the bench. Rest your right knee and shin on the bench. Bend forward and plant your right hand on the bench so that your back's parallel to the floor. Grasp the handle with your left hand, palm facing your body, and pull it back to the starting position: upper arm parallel to the floor and elbow tucked into your side. Inhale as you slowly extend your arm until it's pointing straight behind you. Exhale as you slowly lower the handle to the starting position. Finish your reps, move to the right side of the bench, and shift the bench a few inches to the left of the pulley. Repeat the exercise with your right arm.

Perfect form: Don't jerk the cable back—use a slow, controlled motion. Keep your elbow locked into position during the movement so that your upper arm stays parallel to the floor. Again, your arm is a hinge. Keep your back straight and parallel to the floor. Face forward, not down.

Advanced tip: Remember that good form is much more important than how much weight you lift. The farther you can pull the cable back—the closer you get to full extension of your arm—the better the contraction.

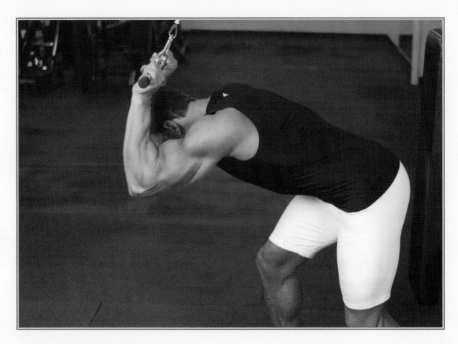

Bent-Over Cable Triceps
Extension—Straight Bar

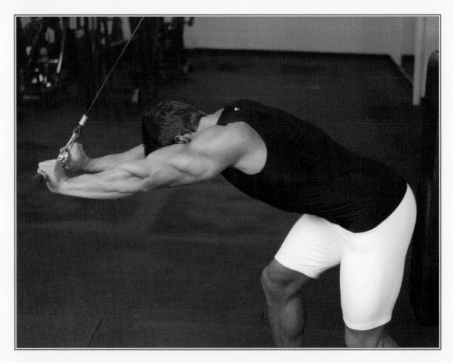

TRICEPS: SECONDARY EXERCISES

Bent-Over Cable Triceps Extension—Straight Bar

(Targets triceps brachii)

Attach a straight bar to a high cable. Facing away from the machine, grasp the bar above your head, with palms facing forward and in a narrow or shoulder-width grip. Pulling the bar forward, lunge ahead with one leg and bend over from the waist to the starting position: torso parallel to the floor. Your upper arms should be extended straight in front of you, also parallel to the floor. Moving only your forearms, inhale as you slowly extend your forearms, pushing the bar forward until your arms are fully extended. Exhale as you slowly move your forearms back to the starting position.

Perfect form: Don't jerk the bar forward—use a slow, controlled motion. Keep your elbow locked into position during the movement so that your upper arm stays parallel to the floor. Again, your arm is a hinge. Keep your back straight and parallel to the floor. Face forward, not down.

Advanced tip: Extend your arms fully to get the best contraction.

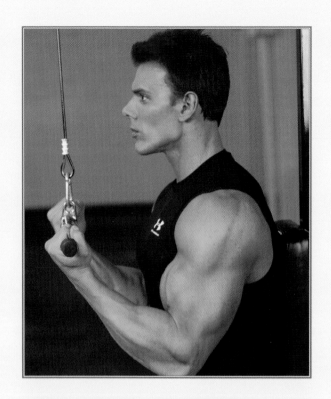

Reverse Grip Cable Pull-Down— Straight Bar

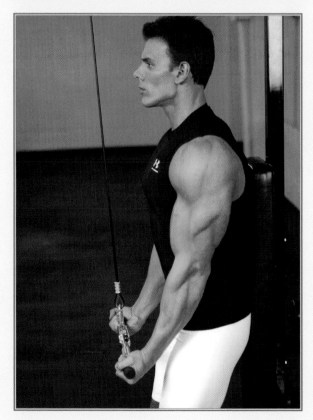

TRICEPS: SECONDARY EXERCISES

Reverse Grip Cable Pull-Down– Straight Bar
(Targets triceps brachii)

Attach a straight bar to a high cable. Stand facing the machine (face away from it if the machine has a backrest for you to use) with knees slightly bent and feet shoulder-width apart. Grasp the bar with palms up, hands shoulder-width apart. Pull the bar down to the starting position: upper arms straight down at your sides, elbows in tight, and forearms extended, holding the bar in front of your chest. Inhale as you use only your forearms to slowly pull the bar down to your thighs, until your arms are fully extended. Exhale as you slowly let the bar curl your forearms back up to your chest.

Perfect form: Don't jerk the bar down—use a slow, controlled motion. Keep your elbow locked at your sides during the movement and your back straight. If the machine has a backrest, use it.

Advanced tip: Step in as close to the machine as you can get while still being able to perform the exercise to increase resistance at the top of the movement.

Variation: To work your triceps separately, try the **One-arm triceps pull-down**: Attach a handle to the high cable and follow the same motion and form.

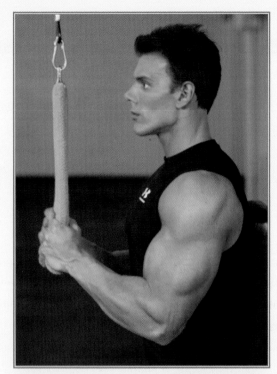

Triceps
Push-Down
—Rope

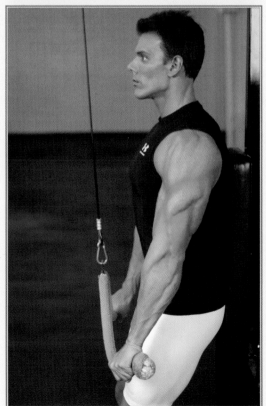

Triceps Push-Down–Rope

(Targets overall triceps)

Attach a rope to a high cable. Stand facing the machine (face away from it if the machine has a backrest for you to use) with knees slightly bent and feet shoulder-width apart. Grasp both ends of the rope with palms facing each other. Pull the rope down to the starting position: upper arms straight down at your sides, elbows in tight, and your forearms extended in front of you parallel to the floor, hands touching. Inhale as you use only your triceps to slowly pull the rope down toward your thighs, until your arms are fully extended. Exhale as you slowly let the rope pull your forearms back up so that they're parallel with the floor.

Perfect form: Don't jerk the rope down—use a slow, controlled motion. Keep your elbow locked at your sides during the movement and your back straight. If the machine has a back-rest, use it. To best isolate your triceps, don't bring your forearms above horizontal at the top of the motion.

Advanced tip: For maximum burn, pull your hands apart and out to the sides at the bottom of the motion and flex your triceps as hard as you can. Be sure to keep your elbows tucked into your side as you do this.

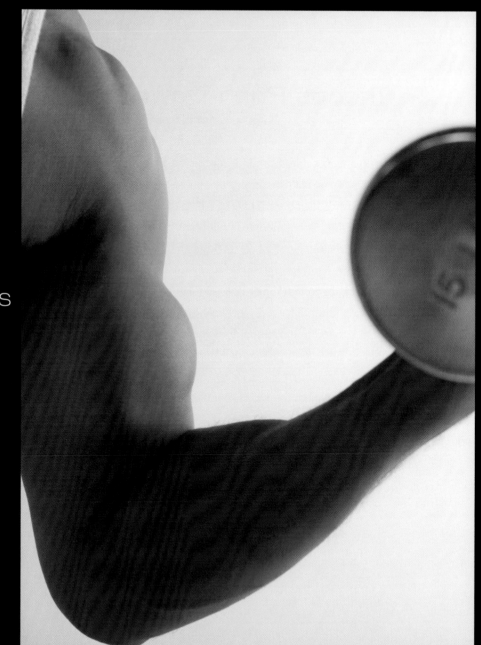

Biceps

Biceps

Without a doubt, the biceps are the most-flexed muscles of all time. Men, women, kids, and grandparents have all flexed their guns in response to the request to "make a muscle." Men have idolized other men with well-developed biceps for years—from the Charles Atlas period to the Arnold Schwarzenegger years to what I like to think of as the Frank Sepe era. And these days, the same goes for women. I wish I had a nickel for every time a woman told me that she wished she had arms like Madonna or Angela Bassett.

Great biceps should have three things: (1) They should be complete, which means they should be fully developed from the elbow to the shoulder; (2) they should have a nice shape—that is, biceps should have a pronounced peak and look more like a basketball player's arm than a football player's arm; and (3) they should have muscle separation—in other words, you should be able to distinguish between your biceps and triceps. There should be a clear division between the two.

You'll be training your biceps by doing curls—lots of curls, all different kinds. The key to good form is to make sure that you keep your biceps isolated to avoid cheating with your chest and shoulders. For most curls, that means keeping your elbows tucked in close to your side throughout the movement. Keep the motion slow, don't rock your body, and don't use momentum.

(**Note:** Except where indicated, all exercises target the entire biceps area.)

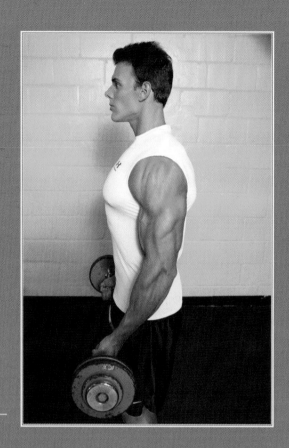

Biceps Curl—
Barbell

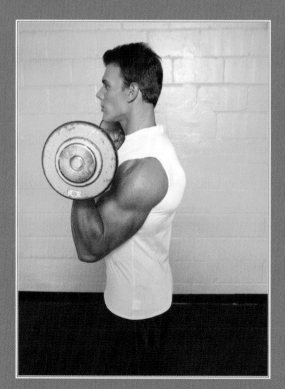

BICEPS: PRIMARY EXERCISES

Biceps Curl–Barbell

Stand with your feet shoulder-width apart and knees slightly bent. Grasp the bar with your palms facing forward and hands shoulder-width apart. Lift the bar from the floor or rack and rest it against your upper thighs, arms fully extended (but elbows not locked). With your elbows pointing straight down and held in tight to your sides, exhale and lift your forearms, slowly curling the bar up toward your chest until your biceps are fully contracted. Inhale as you slowly lower the bar back toward your thighs, elbows still held tightly at your sides.

Perfect form: The key to a good biceps curl is to keep your elbows in place. Don't lift them forward, and don't raise them to the side. Keep your back straight, and don't cheat by rocking your torso back as you lift.

Advanced tip: At the top of your curl, give your biceps an extra tight contraction—just the biceps, not your wrists—to get the most from the exercise.

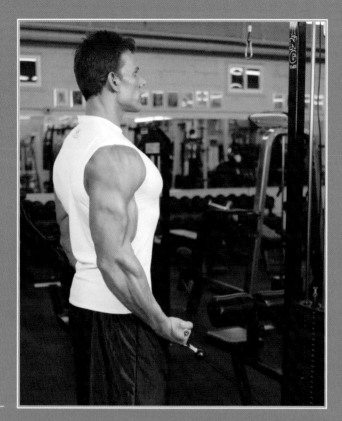

Biceps Curl—
Cable with
Straight Bar

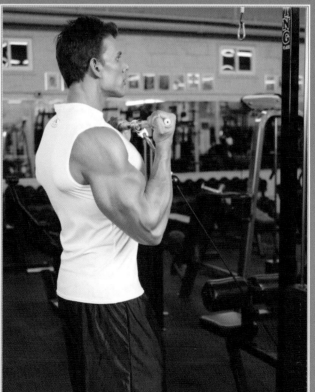

BICEPS: PRIMARY EXERCISES

Biceps Curl–Cable with Straight Bar

Attach a straight bar to the lower pulley of a cable apparatus. Stand one pace back from the pulley, with your feet shoulder-width apart and knees slightly bent. Bend over and grasp the bar with palms facing forward and hands shoulder-width apart. Stand back upright, lifting the bar from the floor until it rests against your upper thighs with arms fully extended (but elbows not locked). With your elbows pointing straight down and held in tight to your sides, exhale and lift your forearms, slowly curling the bar up toward your chest, until your biceps are fully contracted. Inhale as you slowly lower the bar back toward your thighs, elbows still held tightly at your sides.

Perfect form: Keep your elbows in place—don't lift them forward or raise them to the side. Keep your back straight, and don't cheat by rocking your torso back as you lift.

Advanced tip: At the top of your curl, give your biceps an extra tight contraction—just the biceps, not your wrists—to get the most from the exercise.

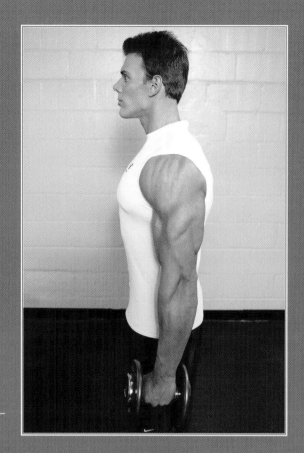

Biceps Curl—
Dumbbell

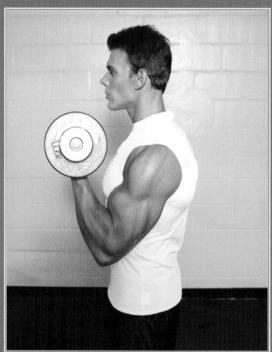

BICEPS: PRIMARY   EXERCISES

Biceps Curl–Dumbbell

Stand with your feet shoulder-width apart and knees slightly bent. Hold a dumbbell in each hand, palms facing each other. With your elbows pointing straight down and held in tight to your sides, inhale and lift your left forearm, slowly curling the dumbbell up toward your chest until your biceps are fully contracted. As you curl the dumbbell up, rotate it so that your palm is facing up at the top of the motion. Exhale as you slowly lower the dumbbell back to your side, rotating it back so that your palm faces your side. Repeat the motion with your right arm.

Perfect form: Keep your elbows locked in place—don't lift them forward or raise them to the side. Keep your back straight, and don't cheat by rocking your torso back as you lift.

Advanced tip: At the top of each curl, give your biceps an extra tight contraction—just the biceps, not your wrist—to get the most from the exercise.

Variation: Try the **Biceps curl–dumbbell** seated on a bench with a backrest to help keep from rocking your torso back as you lift.

Incline
Biceps Curl

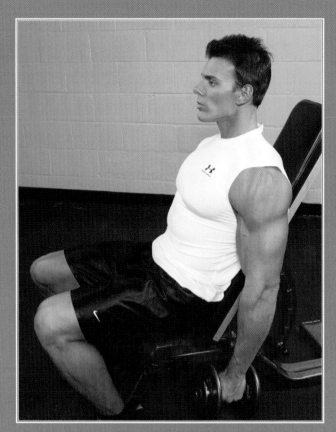

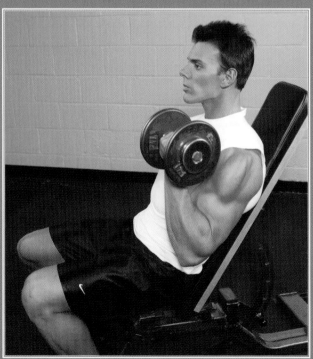

Incline Biceps Curl

Sit on an incline bench with a dumbbell in each hand, palms facing each other and arms hanging straight down at your sides. With your elbows held in tight to your sides, inhale and lift your left forearm, slowly curling the dumbbell up toward your chest until your biceps are fully contracted. As you curl the dumbbell up, rotate it so that your palm is facing up at the top of the motion. Exhale as you slowly lower the dumbbell back to your side, rotating it back so that your palm faces your side. Repeat the motion with your right arm.

Perfect form: To benefit from the inclined position, keep your upper arms pointing straight down throughout the exercise. Keep your elbows in close to your body. Move slowly and don't rock up from the bottom of your curl.

Advanced tip: At the top of each curl, give your biceps an extra tight contraction—just the biceps, not your wrist—to get the most from the exercise.

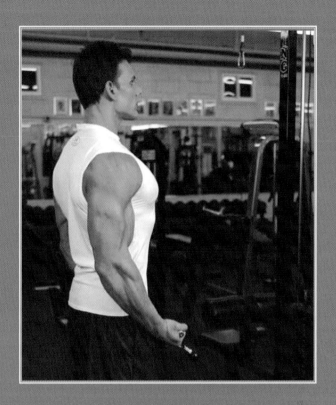

One-Arm
Biceps Curl—
Cable

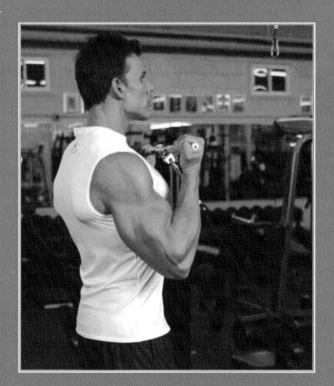

BICEPS: PRIMARY EXERCISES

One-Arm Biceps Curl—Cable

Attach a handle to the lower pulley on a cable apparatus. Stand about a foot from the pulley, feet shoulder-width apart and knees slightly bent. Bend over and grasp the handle with your left hand, palm facing away from you. Stand upright and lift the handle even with your upper thigh, arm fully extended. Place your right hand in the small of your back. Inhale and lift your left forearm, slowly curling the handle up toward your chest until your biceps are fully contracted. Exhale as you slowly lower the handle back to your side. After completing your reps, switch arms, and repeat the exercise with your right arm.

Perfect form: Keep your elbow pointing straight down and tight to your side throughout the exercise.

Advanced tip: At the top of each curl, give your biceps an extra tight contraction—just the biceps, not your wrist—to get the most from the exercise.

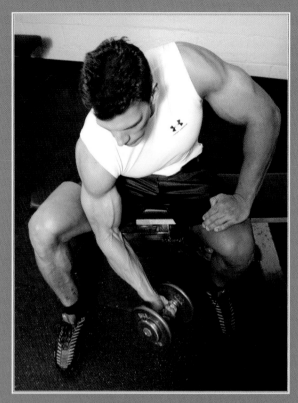

Concentration
Curl—Dumbbell

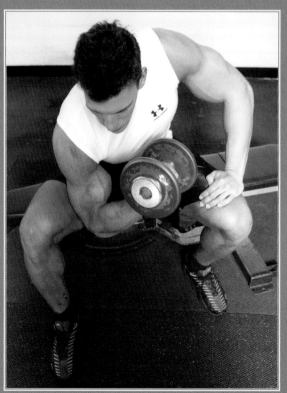

BICEPS: SECONDARY EXERCISES

Concentration Curl–Dumbbell
(Targets upper biceps)

Grab a dumbbell in your left hand and sit on the end of a bench with your feet on the floor, shoulder-width apart. Lean forward slightly and brace your left triceps against the inside of your left thigh. Inhale as you slowly lift the dumbbell up toward your left shoulder. Exhale as you slowly lower the dumbbell until your arm is fully extended. Finish your reps and repeat the exercise with your right arm.

Perfect form: A slight bend forward is all you need—don't rock your back up and down.

Advanced tip: I do this exercise last in my biceps routine to isolate my biceps peak, and I squeeze at the top of the movement as hard as I can.

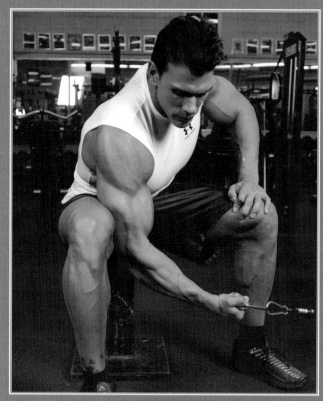

Concentration
Curl—Cable

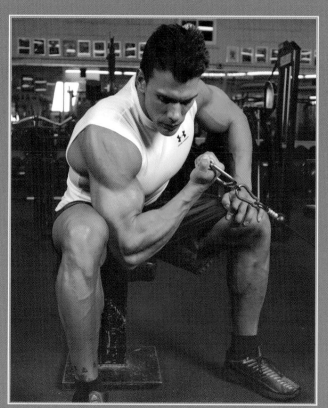

BICEPS: SECONDARY EXERCISES

Concentration Curl—Cable

Attach a handle to a low cable. Position a bench in front of the machine and sit facing it, with your feet shoulder-width apart on the floor. Lean slightly forward, grasp the handle with your left hand (palm facing up), and brace your left triceps against the inside of your left thigh. Inhale as you slowly curl the handle up toward your left shoulder. Exhale as you slowly lower the handle until your arm is fully extended (but your elbows aren't locked). Finish your reps and repeat the exercise with your right arm.

Perfect form: A slight bend forward is all you need. Don't rock your back up and down. And don't jerk the cable up—use a slow, controlled motion.

Advanced tip: Again, squeeze at the top of the movement as hard as you can.

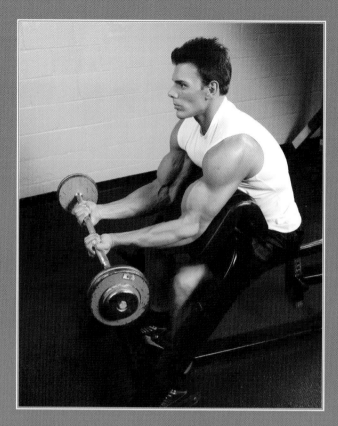

Preacher
Curl—Barbell

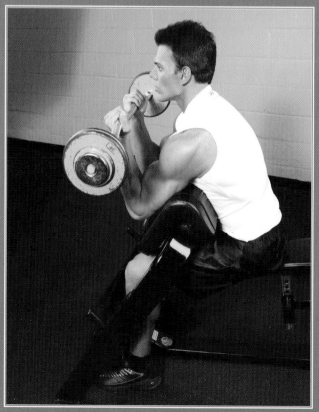

BICEPS: SECONDARY EXERCISES

Preacher Curl–Machine

Adjust the seat height so that when you sit down, the top of the arm pad rests comfortably under your armpits. Brace your triceps against the front of the arm pad, fully extend your arms, and grasp the handles with your palms facing up. Inhale as you slowly curl the handles up toward your shoulders. Exhale as you lower the handles until your arms are fully extended (but elbows aren't locked).

Perfect form: Keep your triceps firmly on the pad throughout the exercise to keep from cheating with your shoulders and chest. Make sure you fully extend your arms to stretch your biceps at the bottom of the motion.

Variation: If your gym doesn't have this machine, use the same motion and form with a preacher bench and barbell to do the **Preacher curl–barbell** exercise (pictured).

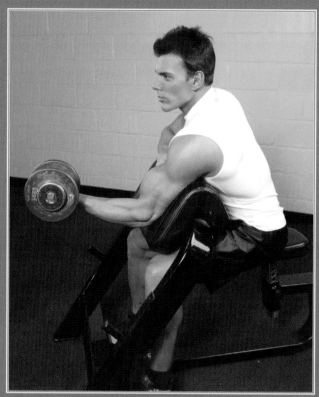

Preacher Curl—
Dumbbell

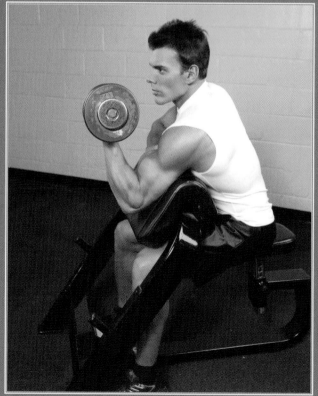

BICEPS: SECONDARY EXERCISES

Preacher Curl–Dumbbell

Adjust the seat height on the preacher bench so that when you sit down, the top of the arm pad rests comfortably under your armpits. Grasp a barbell in your left hand, brace your left triceps against the front of the arm pad, and fully extend your arm. Rest your right arm comfortably over the pad. Inhale as you slowly curl the dumbbell up toward your left shoulder. Exhale as you lower the dumbbell until your arm is fully extended (but your elbow isn't locked). Finish your reps and repeat the exercise with your right arm.

Perfect form: Keep your triceps firmly on the pad throughout the exercise to keep from cheating with your shoulders and chest. Make sure you fully extend your arm to stretch your biceps at the bottom of the motion. Move slowly—don't use momentum.

Advanced tip: I like to do one arm at a time so I can spot myself with the other arm and crank out a few extra reps.

Standing
Hammer
Curl—
Dumbbell

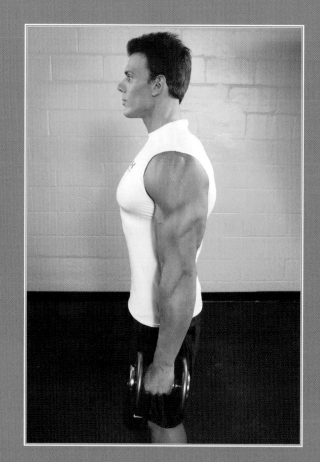

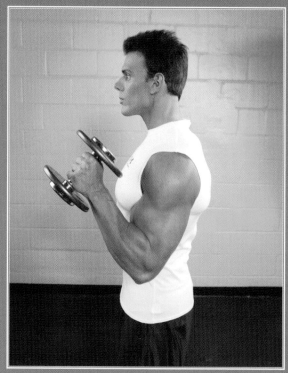

BICEPS: SECONDARY EXERCISES

Standing Hammer Curl—Dumbbell

(Targets lower biceps)

Stand erect, with your legs shoulder-width apart and locked. You should be facing forward with your head up. Grab a pair of dumbbells and hold them at your sides. The dumbbells should be against your outer thighs as your palms face in. Inhale as you curl the dumbbells upward until your forearms touch your biceps. Exhale as you bring the dumbbells back down until your arms are completely extended, while keeping your elbows close to your body.

Perfect form: Keep your elbows close to your side throughout the motion. If you move them out, you're essentially doing a regular biceps curl, *not* a hammer curl. Fully extend your arm to stretch your biceps at the bottom of the motion.

Variation: You can use the same motion and form to do a **Seated hammer curl**.

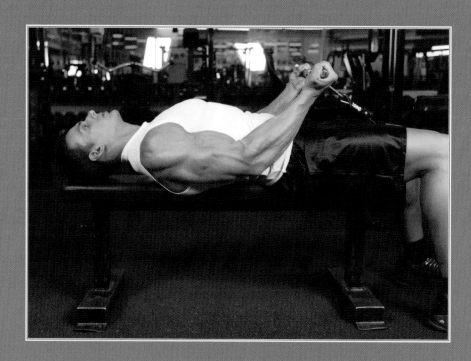

Lying Biceps
Curl—Cable

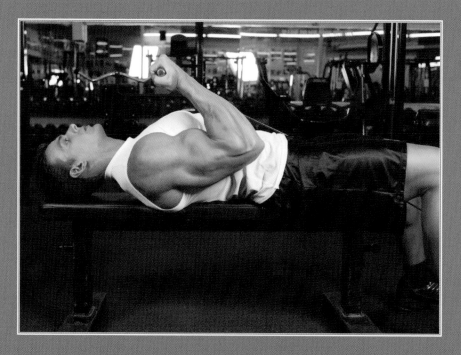

BICEPS: SECONDARY EXERCISES

Lying Biceps Curl–Cable

Attach a straight bar to a cable and position a bench so that it points away from the cable. Sit on the end of the bench, facing the machine, with your feet flat on the floor. Grasp the bar with your hands shoulder-width apart and palms facing up. Lie back flat on the bench, your arms fully extended toward the machine and elbows down at your sides. Inhale as you slowly curl the cable up toward your chest until your biceps are fully contracted. Exhale as you slowly return the bar to the starting position.

Perfect form: Make sure that your elbows are tucked in and your back is flat. Keep your elbows down as you bring the bar toward your chest, as lifting them will weaken your contraction.

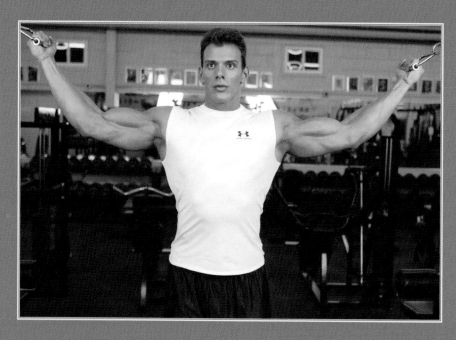

Standing Two-Hand
Overhead Cable Curl

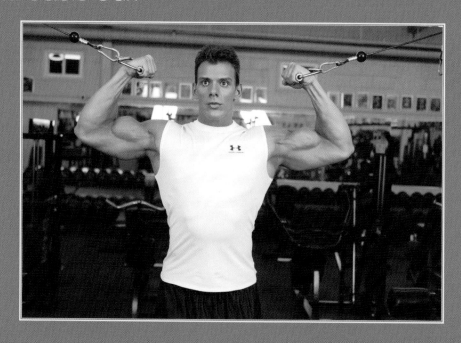

BICEPS: SECONDARY EXERCISES

Standing Two-Hand Overhead Cable Curl

On a twin-cable machine, attach handles to each of the opposing overhead cables. Grasp the left handle in your left hand and the right handle in your right hand (palms facing up). Center yourself between the two weight stacks and stand with your feet shoulder-width apart. Extend your arms out fully to your sides, palms facing up. Inhale as you curl both handles in toward your shoulders, until your biceps are fully contracted. Flex your biceps, and then exhale as you slowly return the handles to the starting position.

Perfect form: Stand up straight, and move nothing but your forearms during the exercise.

Advanced tip: Be careful not to curl your hands forward. You'll get a better contraction if you curl the handles toward the top of your shoulders or even a little behind you.

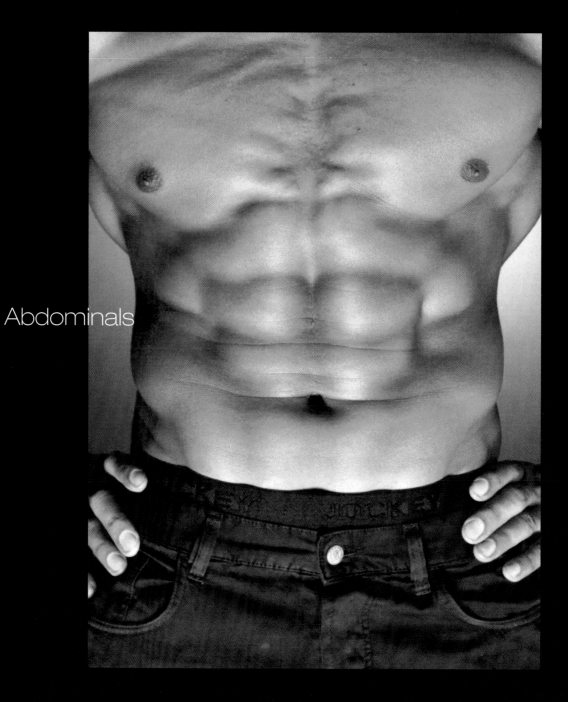

Abdominals

Abdominals

Working your abs won't do any good unless you commit to eating a healthy diet and doing regular cardiovascular exercises, *along with* conscientiously working your abdominal muscles themselves. One of the most discouraging things I see in the gym is when personal trainers have seriously obese people doing tons of sit-ups. Their clients' time would be much better spent on extra cardiovascular work. You need to get rid of the fat before you'll ever see your abs.

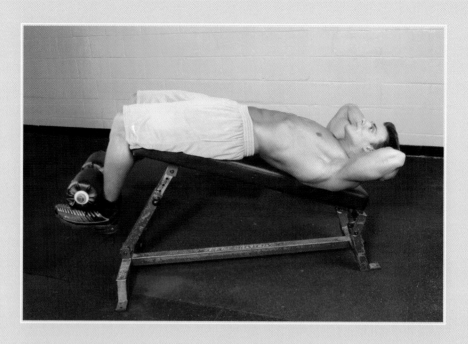

Sit-Up—
Decline Bench

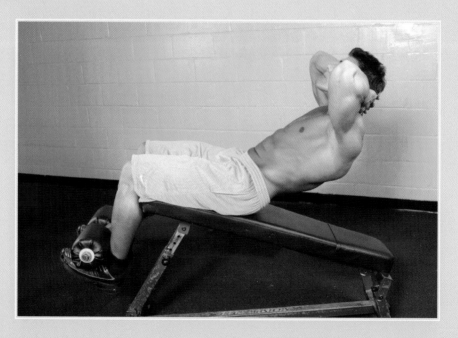

ABDOMINAL   EXERCISES

Sit-Up—Decline Bench

(Targets upper abs)

Lie on your back on a decline bench with your knees up to form a right angle and your feet under the footpads. Place your hands under your head with your fingers loosely laced together. Inhale and slowly contract your abs, curling your head and upper torso up off the board. After your abs have fully contracted, continue to lift up from your hips until your chest comes close to your knees. Exhale as you slowly lower your torso back until your shoulders just touch the bench.

Perfect form: Keep your butt flat on the board. Don't rock, don't pull with your arms, and don't pause at the bottom of the motion.

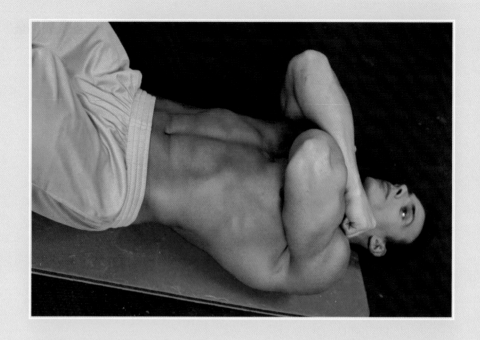

Crunch

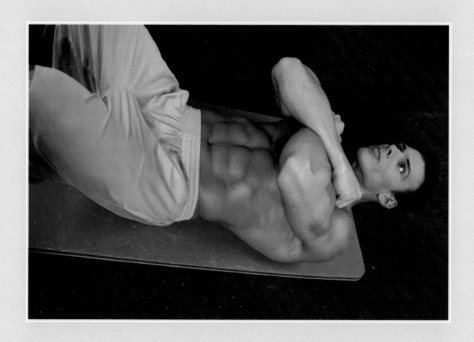

A B D O M I N A L   E X E R C I S E S

Crunch

(Targets upper abs)

Lie on the floor on your back with your knees raised. Keep your feet flat on the floor with your heels near your butt, and fold your hands on your chest. Inhale and slowly contract your abs, curling your head and upper torso up several inches off the floor until your abs are fully contracted. Exhale as you slowly lower your torso back until your shoulders just touch the floor.

Perfect form: Use only your abs. Don't lift your lower back off the floor, don't rock, and don't pause at the bottom of the motion.

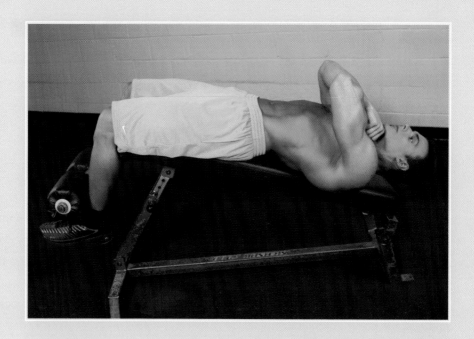

Crunch—Decline Bench or Crunch Board

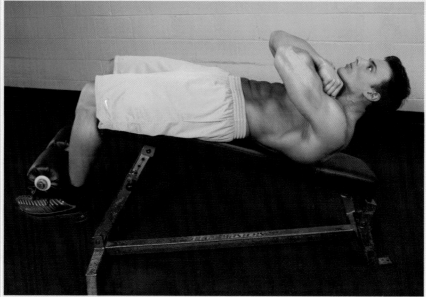

ABDOMINAL   EXERCISES

Crunch—Decline Bench
or Crunch Board
(Targets upper abs)

Lie on your back on a decline bench or crunch board with your knees up, your calves on the calf pad, and your feet under the footpads. Fold your hands on your chest. Inhale and slowly contract your abs, curling your head and upper torso up several inches off the board until your abs are fully contracted. Exhale as you slowly lower your torso back until your shoulders just touch the board.

Perfect form: Keep your lower back flat on the board; your thighs should remain at a right angle to your torso. Use only your abs. Don't rock, and don't pause at the bottom of the motion.

Advanced tip: Many crunch boards or benches can decline so that your head hangs below your hips. Use a declining position to intensify the burn.

Variation: If your gym doesn't have a crunch board, you can perform the exercise by lying on the floor with your calves resting flat on a bench. Keep your thighs at a right angle to your torso.

Crunch—Machine (Variation)
(Targets upper and lower abs)

(Machines will vary.) Sit or lie on the machine with your back firmly against the back pad. Lightly grasp the handles by your ears. Inhale as you curl your shoulders toward your knees, until your abs are fully contracted. Then exhale as you slowly uncurl to the starting position.

Perfect form: Use only your abs—don't pull with your arms or bend at your hips.

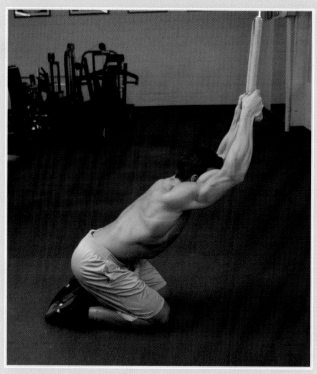

Kneeling
Crunch—Rope

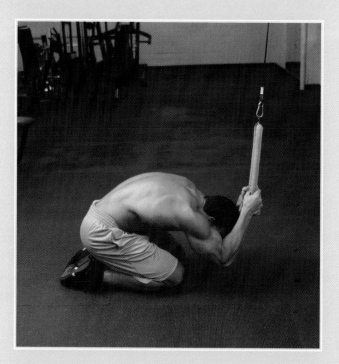

ABDOMINAL   EXERCISES

Kneeling Crunch—Rope

(Targets upper and lower abs)

Attach a rope to an overhead cable. Facing away from the pulley, grasp the two ends of the rope and pull it down behind you to your ears. Kneel down on the ground to the starting position: sitting upright with your butt resting on your heels. Inhale as you slowly pull down on the rope by curling your torso forward until your abs are fully contracted. Exhale as you slowly straighten up to the starting position.

Perfect form: Pull down only with your abs—don't move your hands from next to your ears, bend at your hips, or curl inward.

Seated Crunch—Rope

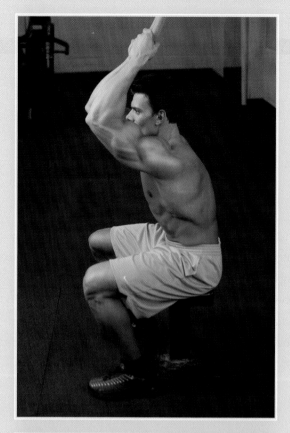

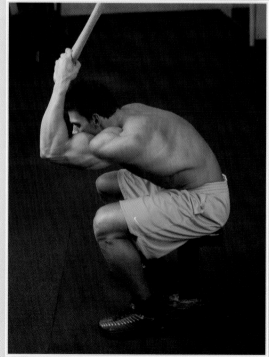

A B D O M I N A L   E X E R C I S E S

Seated Crunch–Rope

(Targets upper and lower abs)

Position a bench a few feet in front of an overhead cable machine. Attach a rope to the cable. Facing away from the pulley, grasp the two ends of the rope and pull it down behind you to your ears. Still facing away from the pulley, sit down on the bench with your feet flat on the floor. Inhale as you slowly pull down on the rope by curling your torso forward until your abs are fully contracted. Exhale as you slowly straighten up.

Perfect form: Pull down only with your abs—don't move your hands from next to your ears or bend at your hips.

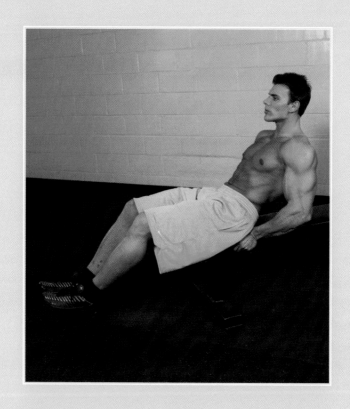

Knee Tuck

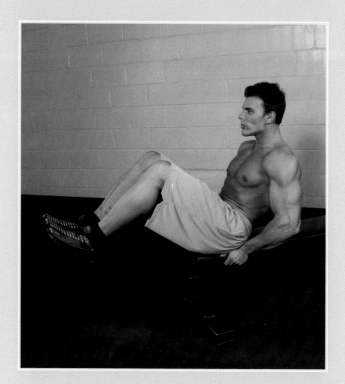

A B D O M I N A L   E X E R C I S E S

Knee Tuck

(Targets upper and lower abs)

Sit on the edge of a flat bench. Lean back slightly and brace your upper body by grasping either side of the bench behind you. Fully extend your legs in front of you. Inhale as you slowly lift your knees up and back toward your chest. Exhale as you lower your knees and extend your legs.

Perfect form: Keep your back straight—don't hunch forward. Move slowly and extend your legs straight out in front of you on each rep.

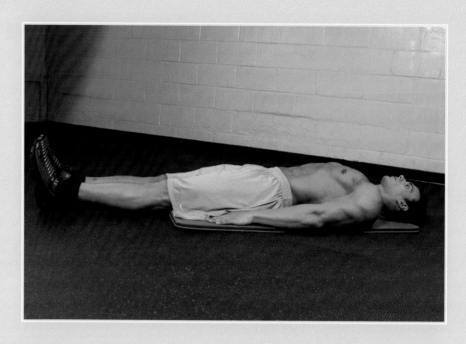

Reverse Crunch or
Lying Leg Raise

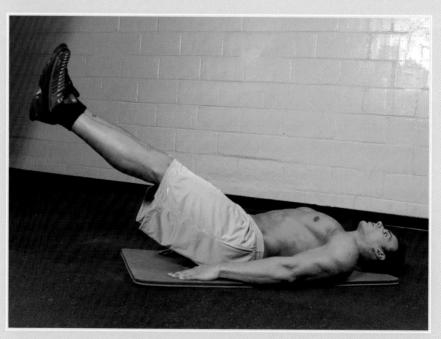

ABDOMINAL   EXERCISES

Reverse Crunch or Lying Leg Raise
(Targets lower abs)

Lie on the floor on your back, with your legs extended and your arms resting at your sides. Inhale and slowly raise your legs to vertical by contracting your abs. Exhale as you slowly lower your legs almost back to the floor.

Perfect form: Use only your abs. Your arms should be relaxed and your lower back shouldn't lift off the floor. Keep continuous tension on your abs, and don't let your feet touch the floor.

Advanced tips: I like to place my hands just under my butt for added stability. I also contract my abs as hard as I can on the way up, pointing my toes to stretch my abs out as much as I can on the way down.

Hanging
Reverse
Crunch

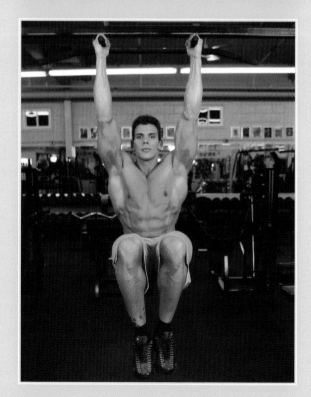

A B D O M I N A L   E X E R C I S E S

Hanging Reverse Crunch

(Targets lower abs**)**

Grasp a chin-up bar with your hands shoulder-width apart, palms facing away from you. Hang from the bar with your arms and legs fully extended (your feet shouldn't touch the floor). Maintaining about a 15-degree angle in your knees, inhale as you slowly pull them up to your chest by contracting your abs. Hold this top position for 2 seconds, then exhale as you slowly lower your legs back to the starting position.

Perfect form: People have a tendency to use momentum to bring their knees up—instead, you should use a slow, continuous motion. *Don't swing.* Keep your knees bent and contract your abs as hard as you can at the top of the motion.

Advanced tips: I like to bring my knees a little farther back at the bottom of the motion because it stretches out my abs nicely. And I recommend that you wrap your wrists to the bar— otherwise your arms might give out before your abs do.

Variation: If hanging from the bar for an entire set is a problem, you can do a **Reverse crunch–vertical bench** exercise (see next page for details on the vertical bench). With your body weight distributed through your arms and shoulders, you may find it easier to concentrate on your abs.

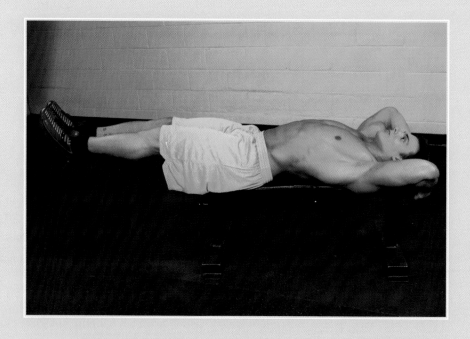

Leg Raise—
Bench

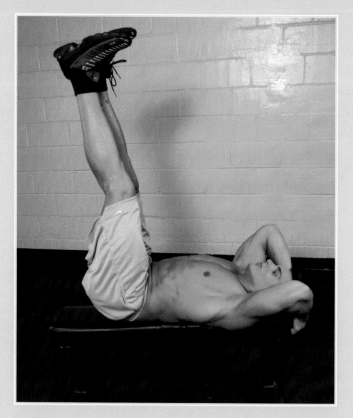

A B D O M I N A L   E X E R C I S E S

Leg Raise–Bench
(Targets lower abs)

Lie flat on your back on a bench with your hips at the bench's end and your legs hanging off. Stabilize yourself by grasping the sides of the bench behind your head. With a slight bend in your knees and your knees and feet together, inhale as you slowly raise your legs up into an L-position. Hold for a second, then exhale as you slowly lower your legs back down to the starting position, hanging straight off the bench.

Perfect form: Nothing moves but your legs—keep your back and butt flat on the bench; don't let your feet touch the floor, and don't swing your legs.

Advanced tip: To intensify the burn, contract your abs as hard as you can at the top of the motion and lower your legs back to the starting position very slowly.

Leg Raise–Vertical Bench (Variation)
(Targets lower abs)

Rest your forearms comfortably on the arm pads, lightly grasp the grips, and press your back flat against the back pad. Shift your weight to your arms as you move your feet off the footrests. With your legs held straight and toes pointed, inhale as you slowly contract your abs and lift your legs up into an L-position. Hold this position for 2 seconds, then exhale as you slowly lower your legs back to the starting position.

Perfect form: Again, momentum is your enemy—don't swing your legs up; keep your back tight against the back pad; and use a smooth, controlled motion. Use only your abs to move only your legs. Keep your legs straight.

Advanced tip: I like to bring my legs up as far as I can—past 90 degrees—to stretch out my abs fully at the bottom and then lift my legs back up really slowly to get a more intense burn.

Variation: Following good form for the hanging reverse crunch (see previous page), you can also perform a **Hanging leg raise.**

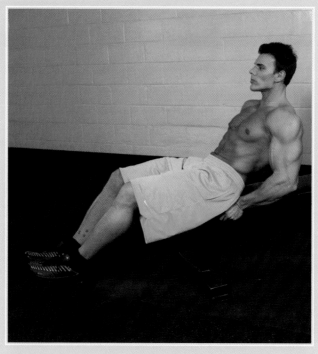

Knee Raise or
Tuck—Flat Bench

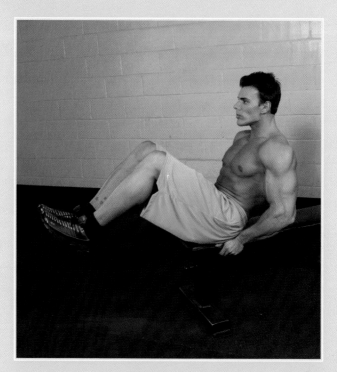

A B D O M I N A L   E X E R C I S E S

Knee Raise or Tuck—Flat Bench
(Targets lower abs)

Sit on the edge of a bench with your feet on the floor. Grasp the sides of the bench on either side of you to stabilize your body. Lean your torso back slightly, lift your feet off the floor, and bend your knees. Your torso and upper legs should form an upright V-shape. Inhale as you slowly bring your knees and chest together. Hold this position for a second and then exhale as you press your chest and knees apart until your feet are just a few inches above the floor (knees still bent).

Perfect form: This is a very simple move once you find a rhythm. Your knees and upper body should move smoothly toward each other, mirroring each other's motion.

Advanced tip: You can increase the intensity of this exercise by extending the range of motion, leaning back as far as you can to widen the V-shape at the starting position.

Frog Kick (Variation)
(Targets lower abs)

Sit sideways on the edge of a bench with your feet on the floor. Grasp the sides of the bench on either side of you to stabilize your body. Lean your torso back slightly, and lift your feet off the floor, keeping your legs straight. Inhale as you slowly bring your knees and chest together over your hips. Hold the position for a second and then exhale as you kick your legs back out straight to the starting position. Your feet shouldn't touch the ground.

Perfect form: Kick your legs out as far as they'll go.

Advanced tip: The contraction of your abs when your knees meet your chest is the key here. Squeeze as hard as you can.

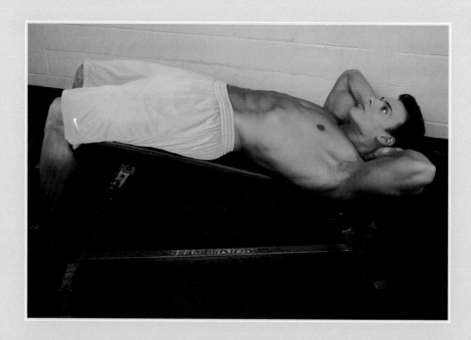

Twisting Crunch—
Decline Bench or
Crunch Board

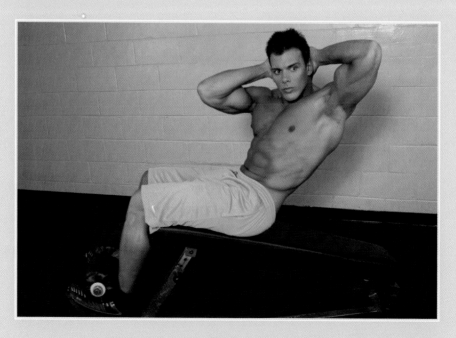

ABDOMINAL   EXERCISES

Twisting Crunch—Decline Bench or Crunch Board
(Targets upper abs and obliques)

Lie on your back on a crunch board with your knees up, your calves on the calf pad, and your feet under the footpads. Fold your hands across your chest and inhale as you contract your abs, slowly raising your shoulders up and toward your chest. Twist your left shoulder up and to the right at the top of the motion. Exhale as you lower your shoulders to the starting position. Finish your reps and then repeat the exercise, this time twisting your right shoulder to the left at the top of the motion.

Perfect form: A slight twist is all you need—overdoing it can injure your back. Keep your hands folded on your chest, your lower back flat on the floor, and your thighs at a right angle to your lower torso. Use a slow, controlled motion—don't pause at the bottom of it.

Advanced tip: Hold the contraction at the top for one second to intensify the burn.

Variation: If your gym doesn't have a crunch board, you can perform the exercise by lying on the floor with your calves resting flat on a bench. Keep your thighs at a right angle to your torso.

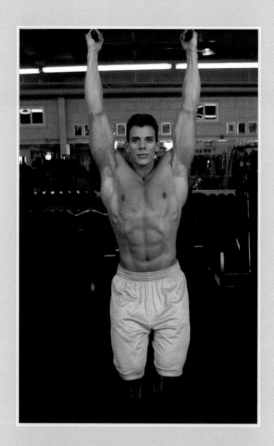

Hanging
Twisting
Leg Raise

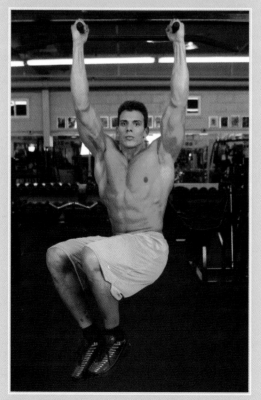

ABDOMINAL   EXERCISES

Hanging Twisting Leg Raise

(Targets obliques)

Grasp a chin-up bar with your hands shoulder-width apart, palms facing away from you. Hang from the bar with your arms and legs fully extended (your feet shouldn't touch the floor). Inhale as you slowly lift your legs (knees slightly bent) up and to the left. Lift your butt at the top of the motion so that your pelvis tilts toward your abs and contracts them hard. Exhale as you slowly lower your legs back to the starting position. Finish your reps, then repeat the exercise, lifting your legs toward the right.

Perfect form: Don't swing your legs up—use a slow, continuous motion.

Advanced tip: As you tilt your pelvis up toward your abs at the top of the motion, go slowly—don't rush the movement. You want to feel the muscles working.

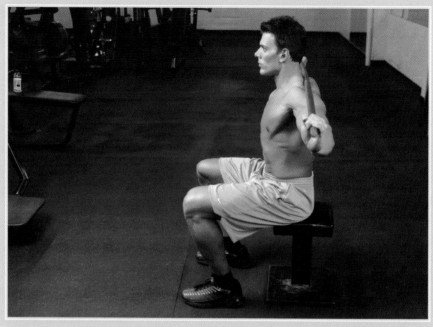

Seated Twist

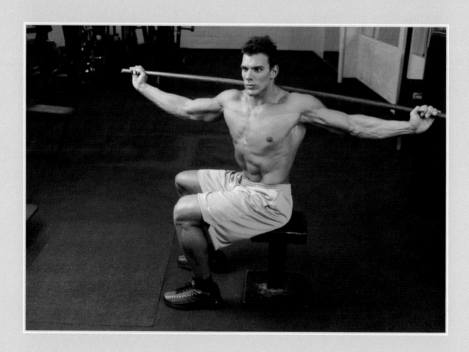

ABDOMINAL   EXERCISES

Seated Twist
(Targets obliques)

Sit on the end of a bench with your feet flat on the floor. Place a lightweight pole or tube behind your neck, resting across your shoulders. Extend your arms straight out to your sides and hang your hands over the ends of the pole. Exhale as you slowly twist your shoulders to the left and then inhale as you twist them to the right.

Perfect form: Restrict the motion to your arms and shoulders. Your hips and lower body should be motionless.

Advanced tip: Most people want toned obliques, not bigger ones. Unless your body is totally ripped, large obliques can make you look fat. Avoid using weight for twists unless you actually want to build your obliques.

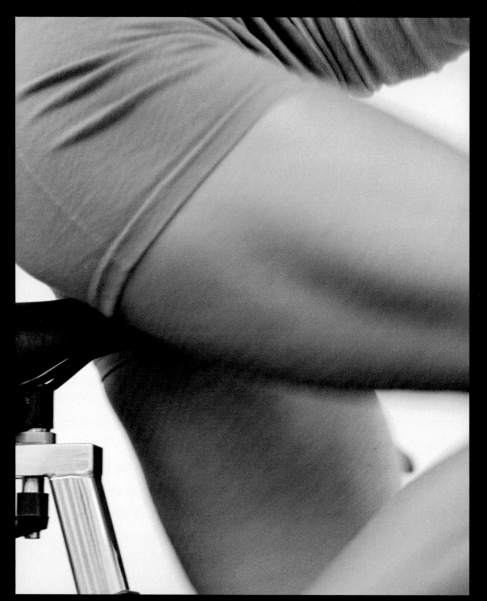

Upper
Legs

Upper Legs

Growing up, I had what people called "bird legs." I used to wear two pairs of sweatpants to the gym so that my legs would appear thicker. You could have painted my legs silver and used them as kickstands for bicycles—they were that skinny. Needless to say, I came to love training my legs.

Learn to build and use your legs. Doing so will spare your back and make essential everyday activities such as walking and climbing stairs easier *and* more useful. Using more muscle mass to do these things will increase your metabolism—in fact, you'll burn more calories with every step you take.

The three major muscles you work when you exercise your upper legs are the quadriceps or "quads" (front thigh), hamstrings (rear thigh), and glutes (butt). Whatever level you're working on, I strongly recommend that you do at least one squatting exercise because they build the entire leg. Squats are without a doubt the best way to tone and strengthen the quads, hamstrings, and calves. I feel that they're also the best for building a firm backside. So if you really want to get ride of some of that junk in your trunk, don't be afraid to squat. As many bodybuilders say, "Squat or rot!"

Legs should be trained with the same intensity as all of your other body parts. Be sure to breathe correctly and to use good form. And remember this: If you're thinking about skipping a leg day, you can't and won't build a great body. As I mentioned previously, any sturdy structure must be solidly built from the ground up.

(**Note:** Except where indicated, these exercises target the entire upper leg/butt region.)

Squat—
Barbell

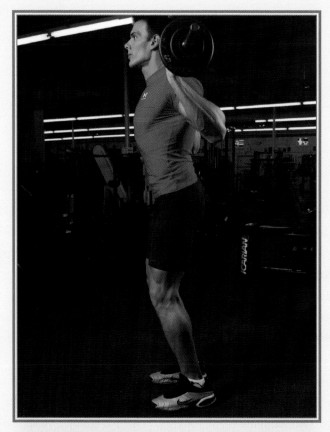

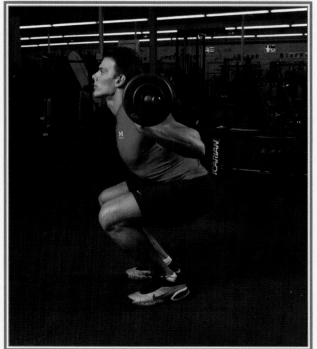

UPPER LEGS: PRIMARY EXERCISES

Squat–Barbell

Start with a loaded bar, which should be just below your shoulder height on a squat rack. Grasp the bar with palms facing down and a wide grip, and duck your head under the bar so that it's resting comfortably across your shoulders. Step forward, placing your feet shoulder-width apart directly below the bar. With your back arched slightly, press up from your thighs and butt, straightening your legs (keep your knees slightly bent) and lifting the bar off the rack. Step back from the rack to the starting position: shoulders back, lower back slightly arched, and the weight of the bar squarely over your feet. Inhale as you bend at the knees and hips, slowly lowering your butt back and behind you until your thighs are parallel to the floor. Exhale as you slowly press back up to the starting position.

Perfect form: The bar should rest behind your neck, not on it—that is, its weight should be on your shoulders. As you lower the weight, move your knees forward toward, but not past, your toes. As you drop your butt back, keep your shoulders up and squarely over your feet. Look straight ahead, not down. The bar should move straight up and down, not forward or back. Maintain a slight arch in your lower back throughout the move, but don't use your back to lift the weight—use only your legs and butt. To avoid injuring your knees, your thighs should never drop below horizontal.

Advanced tip: Push from your heels, not the balls of your feet.

Variations: For greater safety, or just to practice the squat motion, try a **Squat–Smith machine**: Follow the same motion and form with a Smith machine instead of a regular barbell. This will guarantee that the bar moves only straight up and down. If you have weak or injury-prone knees, try a **Half squat** using either a barbell or a Smith machine: Follow the same motion and form, but don't drop your butt all the way down to the point that your thighs are parallel to the floor. You should do half squats extra slowly to compensate for the decreased range of motion.

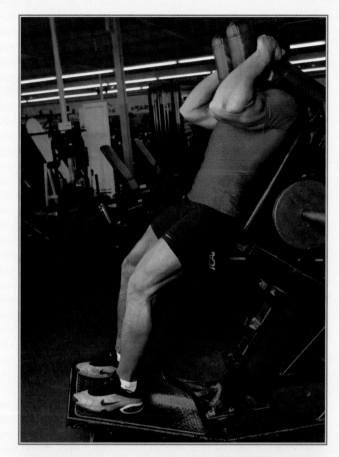

Squat—
Machine

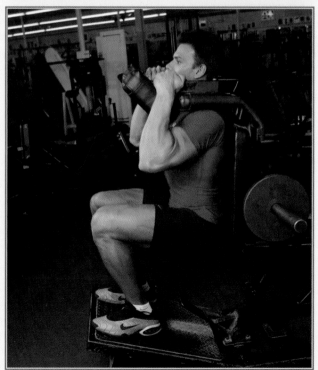

Squat–Machine

(Machines will vary.) Plant your shoulders under the shoulder pads and lightly grasp the handles. Step onto the footplate, making sure that your feet are shoulder-width apart and directly below your shoulders. With your back arched slightly, press up from your thighs and butt, straightening your legs (keep your knees slightly bent) and lifting the shoulder pads off the rest to the starting position. Disengage the rest. Keeping your shoulders back and a slight arch in your lower back, inhale as you bend at the knees and hips, slowly lowering your butt back and behind you until your thighs are parallel to the footplate. Exhale as you slowly press back up to the starting position.

Perfect form: As you lower the weight, move your knees forward toward, but not past, your toes. As you drop your butt back, keep your shoulders up. Look straight ahead, not down. Maintain a slight arch in your lower back throughout the move, but don't use your back to lift the weight—use only your legs and butt. To avoid injuring your knees, your thighs should never drop below parallel to the footplate.

Advanced tip: Push from your heels, not the balls of your feet.

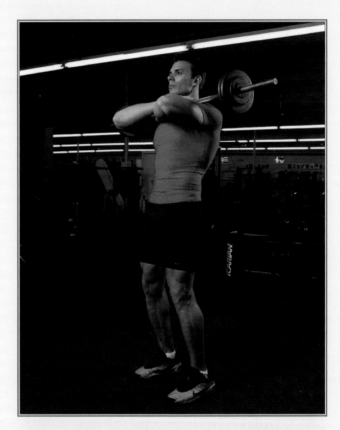

Front Squat
—Barbell

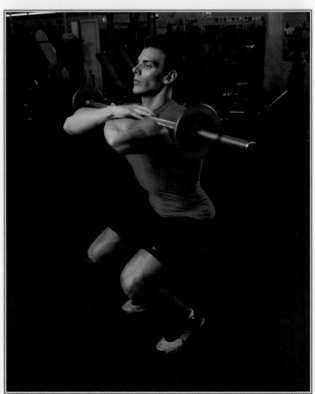

UPPER LEGS: PRIMARY EXERCISES

Front Squat–Barbell

Start with a loaded bar, which should be just below your shoulder height on a squat rack. Step under the bar so that it's resting squarely on your upper chest and shoulders. Cross your arms in front of your chest and grasp the bar at your shoulders. Step forward, placing your feet shoulder-width apart and directly below the bar. With your back arched slightly, press up from your thighs and butt, straightening your legs (keep your knees slightly bent) and lifting the bar off the rack. Step back from the rack to the starting position: shoulders back, lower back slightly arched, and the weight of the bar squarely over your feet. Inhale as you bend at the knees and hips, slowly lowering your butt back and behind you until your thighs are parallel to the floor. Exhale as you slowly press back up to the starting position.

Perfect form: As you lower the weight, move your knees forward toward, but not past, your toes. As you drop your butt back, keep your shoulders up and squarely over your feet. Look straight ahead, not down. The bar should move straight up and down, not forward or back. Maintain a slight arch in your lower back throughout the move, but don't use your back to lift the weight—use only your legs and butt. To avoid injuring your knees, your thighs should never drop below horizontal.

Advanced tip: Push from your heels, not the balls of your feet.

Variation: For greater safety, or just to practice the squat motion, try a **Front squat–Smith machine**: Follow the same motion and form with a Smith machine instead of a regular barbell. This will guarantee that the bar moves only straight up and down.

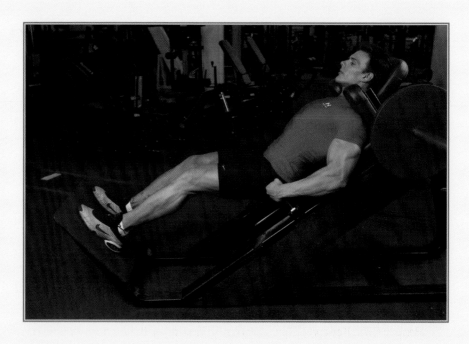

Hack Squat—
Machine

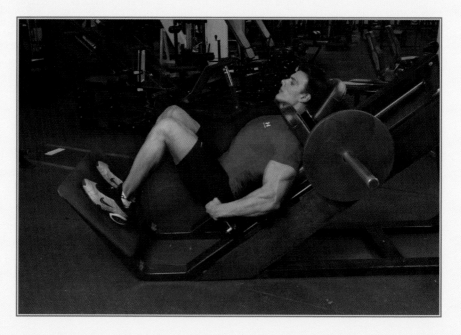

UPPER LEGS: PRIMARY EXERCISES

Hack Squat–Machine

Step into the hack machine and plant your shoulders squarely under the shoulder pads. With your head and back flat against the backrest, place your feet on the footplate, positioning them shoulder-width apart somewhere between the middle and top of the plate. Lift the shoulder pads off their rest and straighten your legs (keeping your knees slightly bent). Disengage the rest. Slowly inhale as you lower the weight until your thighs are parallel to the footplate. Exhale as you slowly press the weight back up.

Perfect form: Keep your head and back firmly against the backrest throughout the exercise. The hack squat can be rough on the knees, so don't let them move ahead of your toes at any point. Move slowly and stop at any sign of knee pain or stress.

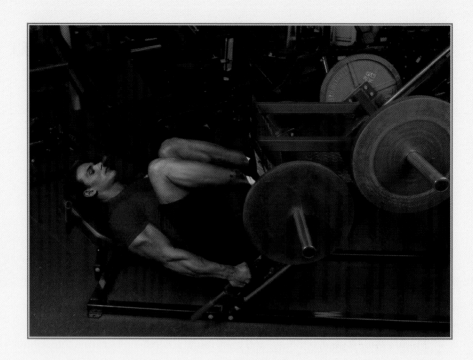

Leg Press—
Machine

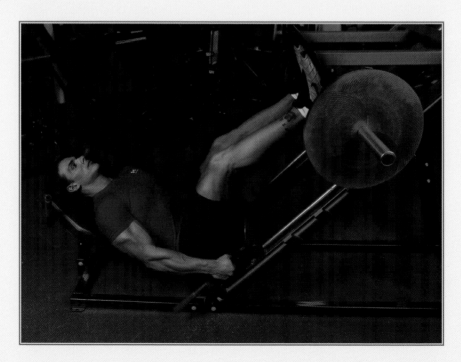

UPPER LEGS: PRIMARY EXERCISES

Leg Press–Machine

Adjust the angle of the backrest so that you're comfortable with your knees pulled up close to your chest. Sit in the machine with your head and the small of your back firmly against the backrest. Plant your feet shoulder-width apart on the footplate. Lift the footplate off its rest and straighten your legs (keeping your knees slightly bent). Disengage the rest. Inhale as you slowly lower the weight until your knees are close to your chest. Exhale as you slowly press the weight back up.

Perfect form: Keep the small of your back against the backrest throughout the exercise. Arching off the backrest as you lower the weight can cause back injury.

Advanced tip: Try doing single-leg sets every once in a while to make sure both of your legs are equally strong.

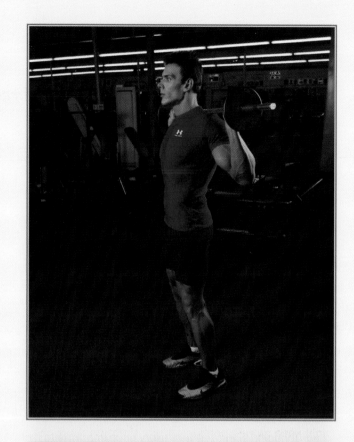

Lunge—
Barbell

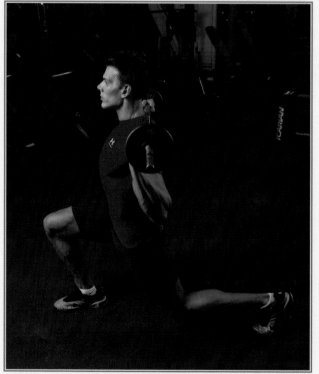

Lunge–Barbell

Start with a loaded bar, which should be just below your shoulder height on a squat rack. Grasp the bar with palms down and a wide grip. Duck your head under the bar so that it's resting comfortably across your shoulders, and step forward, placing your feet shoulder-width apart directly below the bar. With your back arched slightly, press up from your thighs and butt, straightening your legs (keep your knees slightly bent) and lift the bar off the rack. Step back far from the rack to the starting position: back straight and shoulders directly above hips. Inhale as you take a large step forward with your left foot. Once your foot is planted, continue to lunge forward, your left knee moving ahead until it's just above your toes. Your right heel will lift off the floor as your right knee moves toward the floor. Press back off your left foot and return to the starting position with your feet shoulder-width apart under the bar. Repeat the exercise with your right leg. Alternate legs until your set is complete.

Perfect form: The bar should rest behind your neck, not on it—that is, its weight should be on your shoulders. Keep your back straight and your shoulders back and directly above your hips throughout the exercise. Look straight ahead, not down. As you lunge forward, extend your knee until it's just above your toes, no farther.

Advanced tip: To get the best stretch out of your lunges, focus on the drop. Slowly bring the knee of your rear leg as close to the floor as you can.

Variation: For easier balancing, try the **Lunge–dumbbell**: Instead of the barbell, hold a dumbbell in each hand with your arms straight down at your sides and follow the same motion and form.

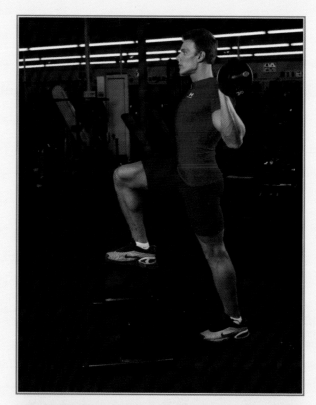

Step-Up—
Barbell

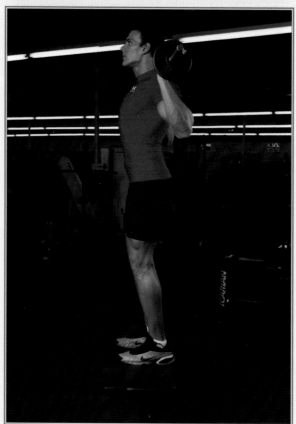

UPPER LEGS: PRIMARY EXERCISES

Step-Up–Barbell

Start with a loaded bar, which is just below your shoulder height on a squat rack. Grasp the bar with palms down and a wide grip and duck your head under the bar so that it's positioned comfortably across your shoulders. Step forward, placing your feet shoulder-width apart directly below the bar. With your back arched slightly, press up from your thighs and butt, straightening your legs (keep your knees slightly bent) and lifting the bar off the rack. Step back from the rack and move to face a flat bench in the starting position: back straight and shoulders directly above your hips. Place your left foot on the bench, then inhale as you step onto the bench with your right foot and stand up straight. Exhale as you step back off the bench with your right foot and then move your left foot back to the starting position on the floor. Switch legs and repeat the exercise. Alternate legs until your set is complete.

Perfect form: The bar should rest behind your neck, not on it—that is, its weight should be on your shoulders. Keep your back straight and your shoulders back and directly above your hips throughout the exercise. Look straight ahead, not down.

Variation: For easier balancing, try the **Step-up–dumbbell**: Instead of the barbell, hold a dumbbell in each hand with your arms straight down at your sides and follow the same motion and form.

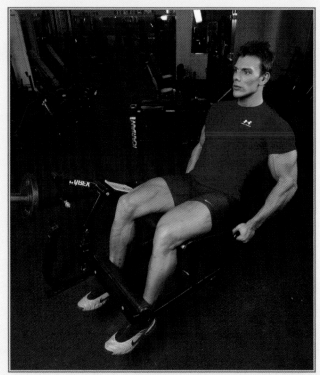

Leg Extension—
Machine

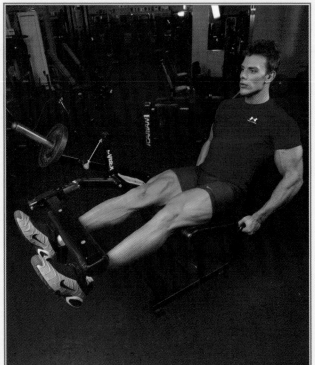

UPPER LEGS: SECONDARY EXERCISES

Leg Extension—Machine
(Targets quads)

(Machines will vary.) Adjust the backrest so that when your back is flat against it, your knees are just beyond the seat and even with the leg bar's axis of motion. Adjust the shin pad so that it rests comfortably just above your ankles. Sit in the machine with your back flush against the backrest and your shins behind the shin pad. If there are handles at your sides, lightly grasp them. Point your toes outward and inhale as you slowly lift your ankles, lifting the shin pad until your legs are fully extended (but knees aren't locked). Exhale as you slowly lower the shin pads to the starting position.

Perfect form: Use a slow, controlled motion—don't lift your butt up off the seat or move your upper body during this exercise. Let your legs do the work.

Advanced tips: At the top of the motion, pause for a second and squeeze your quadriceps as hard as you can for a killer burn. Try doing single-leg sets every once in a while to make sure that both of your legs are equally strong.

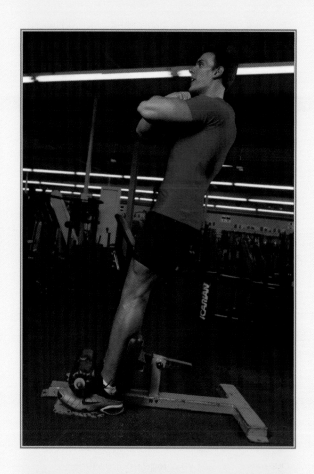

Braced
Squat

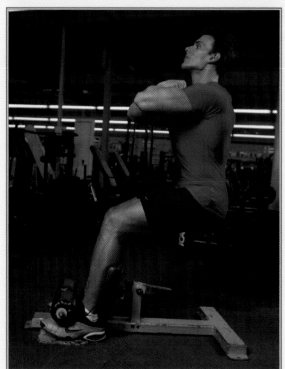

UPPER LEGS: SECONDARY EXERCISES

Braced Squat
(Targets quads)

Stand facing a stable, heavy machine or racked bar with your feet shoulder-width apart. Tightly grasp the machine or bar at hip level with your stronger arm (whichever hand you write with) as you hold a plate tightly to your chest with your other arm. Keeping your shoulders back, a slight arch in your lower back and the weight of the plate squarely over your feet, inhale as you bend at the knees and hips, slowly lowering your butt back and behind you until your thighs are parallel to the floor or as low as you can go. Allow your heels to lift off the floor as you drop. Exhale as you slowly press back up to a standing position, your heels lowering to the floor.

Perfect form: As you drop your butt back, keep your shoulders up and squarely over your feet. Look straight ahead, not down. As you drop, move your knees forward toward, but not past, your toes. Your shoulders should move straight up and down, not forward or back. Maintain a slight arch in your lower back throughout the move, but don't use your back to lift the weight. Use only your legs and butt.

Advanced tip: Form is very important here, so don't use a weight you can't handle. Make sure that the machine or bar you're holding on to can support you and the plate you're clutching, otherwise you'll find yourself flat on the floor with a weight lying on your chest.

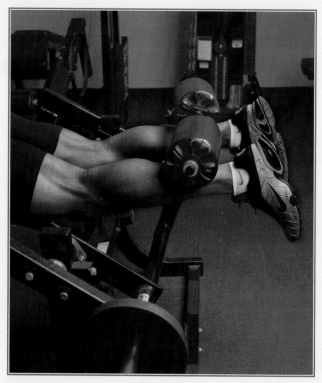

Lying Hamstring
Curl—Machine

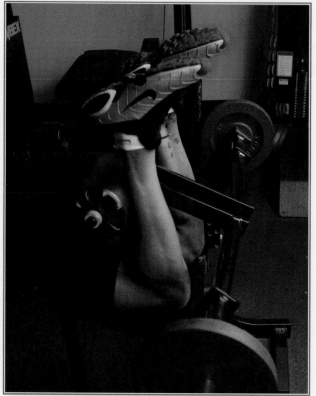

UPPER LEGS: SECONDARY EXERCISES

Lying Hamstring Curl—Machine
(Targets hamstrings)

Adjust the leg bar so that when your knees are even with the machine's axis of motion, the calf pad rests just above your ankles. Lie face down on the machine (if it has handles, lightly grasp them) and plant your calves firmly under the calf pad. Inhale as you slowly curl your ankles up until the leg bar touches the back of your hamstrings. Exhale as you slowly lower the leg bar back to the starting position.

Perfect form: This exercise will do you no good if you lift your hips off the pad. Concentrate on keeping your lower abs tight and your hips flat against the pad. Curl the bar up as far as you can on every rep. A full range of motion is critical.

Advanced tips: To guarantee that I keep my hips down, I use my arms to press my chest and shoulders up several inches off the bench. That makes cheating almost impossible. Also, try doing single-leg sets every once in a while to make sure that both of your legs are equally strong.

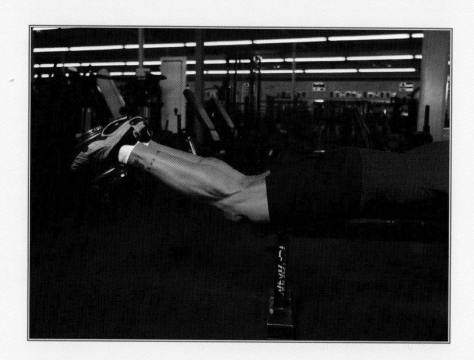

Prone Hamstring
Curl—Dumbbell

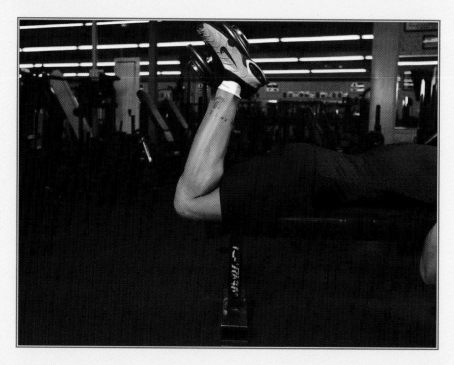

UPPER LEGS: SECONDARY EXERCISES

Prone Hamstring Curl–Dumbbell

(Targets hamstrings)

Stand a dumbbell on end on the floor, a foot or so from the end of a bench. Lie facedown, with your knees just off the end of the bench near the dumbbell. Grasp the dumbbell's grip between your feet so that the top of it rests on your soles. (It helps to have a spotter lift the dumbbell and place it securely between your feet.) Make sure the dumbbell is secured. Inhale as you slowly curl the dumbbell up toward your hamstrings, as far as you can go. Exhale as you slowly lower the dumbbell until your legs are fully extended (but knees aren't locked).

Perfect form: Concentrate on keeping your lower abs tight and your hips flat against the pad. Don't lift them.

Advanced tips: You can increase the difficulty of this exercise by performing it on a long incline board, positioning your knees just above where the board meets the floor. Since you probably have a spotter to get the dumbbell securely between your feet here, you might as well make good use of him or her. When you near the end of your set and your hamstrings are fatigued, have him or her help you lift the dumbbell all the way up and then slowly lower it back down yourself. Crank out those extra reps!

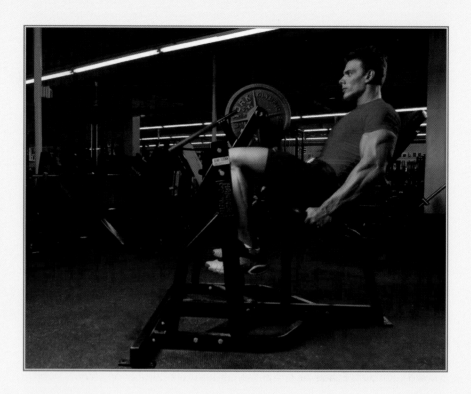

Seated Hamstring
Curl—Machine

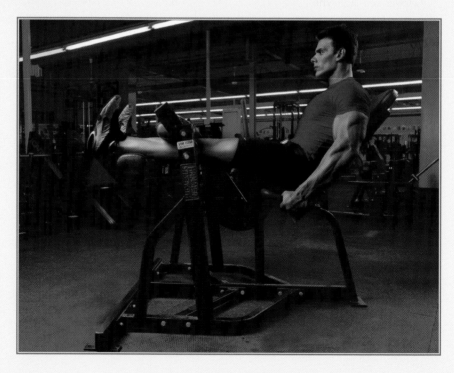

UPPER LEGS: SECONDARY EXERCISES

Seated Hamstring Curl—Machine

(Targets hamstrings)

(Machines will vary.) Adjust the backrest so that when your back is flat against it, your knees are just beyond the seat and even with the leg bar's axis of motion. Adjust the calf pad so that your lower calves rest on top of it. Sit in the machine with your back flush against the backrest and your calves against the calf pad. If there's a thigh pad, bring it down tight against your thighs. If there are handles at your sides, lightly grasp them. Inhale as you slowly curl the leg bar back toward your butt. Exhale as you slowly let the bar return to the starting position.

Perfect form: Keep your back against the backrest. Momentum is your enemy, so don't swing the your legs back and forth. Use a very slow, controlled motion.

Advanced tip: When you've curled your feet back as far as they can go, squeeze your hamstrings tightly and hold the position for two seconds.

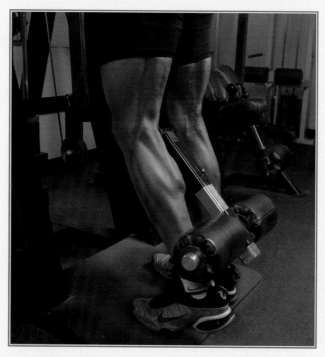

Standing Hamstring
Curl—Machine

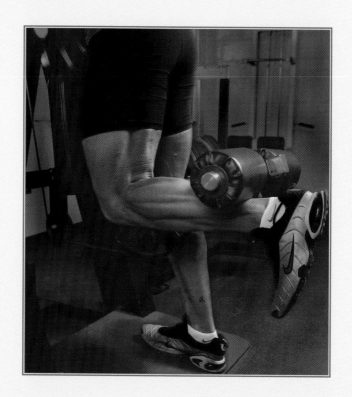

UPPER LEGS: SECONDARY EXERCISES

Standing Hamstring Curl—Machine
(Targets hamstrings)

(Machines will vary.) Lift your right knee onto the elevated kneepad, and plant the bottom of your left calf against the calf pad. Lean forward and plant your forearms on the arm pads. Lightly grasp the handles. Inhale as you slowly curl your left ankle back and up toward your hamstring, as far as you can go. Contract your left hamstring and hold this position for a second at the top of the motion. Exhale as you slowly lower your left foot back to the starting position. Repeat with your right leg.

Perfect form: Curl the pad up as far as you can go, then lower it all the way back down again. Use the fullest range of motion and eliminate momentum.

Advanced tip: A super-slow motion will yield dramatic results.

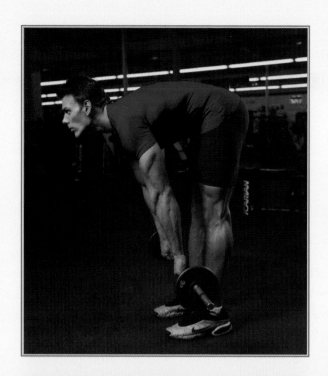

Stiff-Legged
Dead Lift—
Barbell

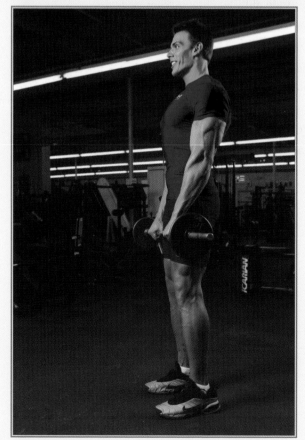

UPPER LEGS: SECONDARY EXERCISES

Stiff-Legged Dead Lift–Barbell
(Targets hamstrings and gluts)

Lift a barbell off a rack with an overhand grip, hands shoulder-width apart. Stand with your feet shoulder-width apart and your knees locked, the bar resting against your thighs, your arms fully extended. With your back straight, bend forward from the waist to the starting position, with your upper body parallel to the floor. The barbell should be hanging at arm's length below your shoulders. Keeping your knees locked, inhale as slowly lift your torso and stand up straight, the bar hanging in front of your upper thighs. Exhale as you slowly bend forward and lower your torso back to parallel with the floor.

Perfect form: Don't bend your knees—bend forward at the waist.

Advanced tip: If you can lower the barbell down so far that it touches the floor (easy with larger plates), stand on a step—a block of wood, several stacked plates, even a bench—to do the exercise. That way, you'll get a full extension at the bottom of the motion.

Variation: You can also try a **Stiff-legged dead lift–dumbbell**: Instead of the bar, hold a dumbbell in each hand and follow the same motion and form.

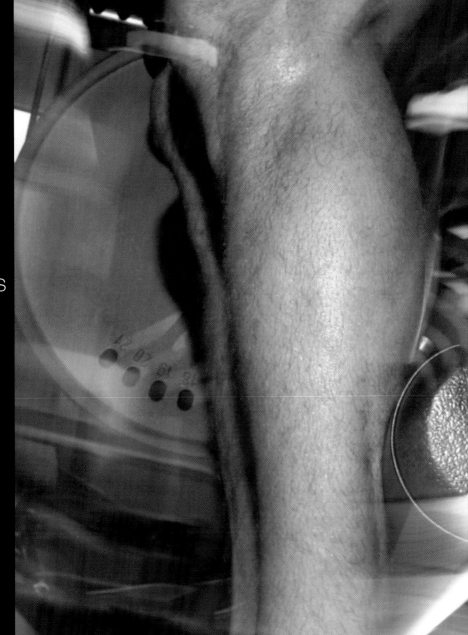

alves

Calves

How many times have you been at the beach and seen someone with a mostly fantastic body—that is, someone who looks like a superhero from their shoulders down to their knees . . . and then resembles a flamingo from the knees down? It just goes to show that people shouldn't neglect their calves.

Building your body starts from the ground up. Every skyscraper needs a strong foundation—the same goes for your body. If you want a well-proportioned physique, then you'd better train your calves.

Calves are worked indirectly when you perform most leg exercises, especially squats, lunges, and leg presses. Unfortunately, indirect exercise isn't enough to build great calves. You have to target your calves specifically because these muscles need a lot of stimulation in order to get them to grow.

I can honestly tell you that it was extremely hard for me to develop any sort of mass in my calves. When I started working out, I had some of the skinniest legs you've ever seen. But through a lot of hard work, I brought my calves up to a respectable level of development that's more or less consistent with that of the rest of my body.

A lot of people are genetically blessed with muscular calves. If you're not one of the lucky ones, you'll need to stay consistent, pay attention to your form, and train very intensely. The following exercises will help mold your entire calf region.

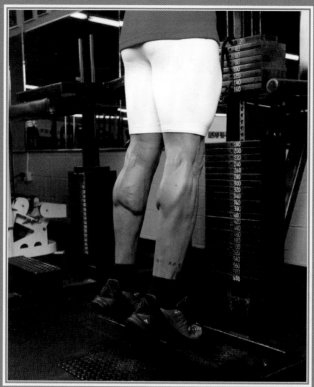

Standing Calf
Raise—Machine

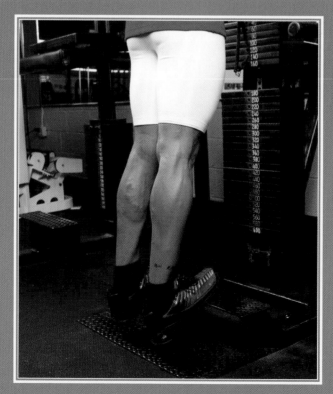

CALVES EXERCISES

Standing Calf Raise—Machine

Place your shoulders under the shoulder pads and lightly grasp the handles. Place the balls of your feet flat on the footplate, shoulder-width apart. Lift the shoulder pad as you straighten your legs, keeping your knees slightly bent. Inhale as you press up from your toes, slowly lifting your heels as high as you can above the level of the footplate. Then exhale as you slowly lower your heels as far down below the footplate as you can.

Perfect form: Keep your knees slightly bent, and lift only with your calves. Don't press from your thighs.

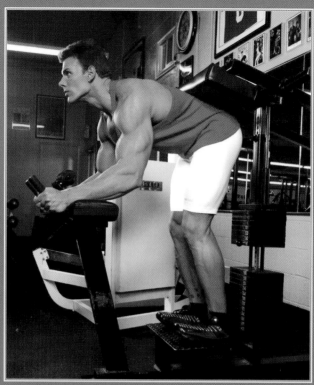

Donkey Calf
Raise—Machine

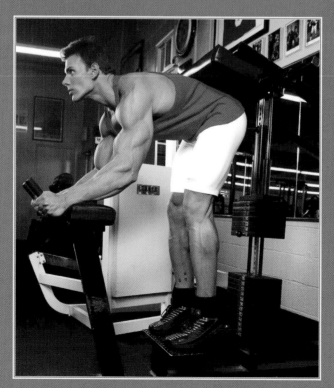

Donkey Calf Raise—Machine

Rest your forearms on the arm pad and lightly grasp the handles as you slide the small of your back under the back pad. Press the back pad up as you place the balls of your feet flat and shoulder-width apart on the footplate. Straighten your legs, keeping your knees slightly bent. Inhale as you press up from your toes, slowly lifting your heels as high as you can above the level of the footplate. Then exhale as you slowly lower your heels down as far below the footplate as you can.

Perfect form: Keep your knees slightly bent, and lift only with your calves. Don't press from your thighs.

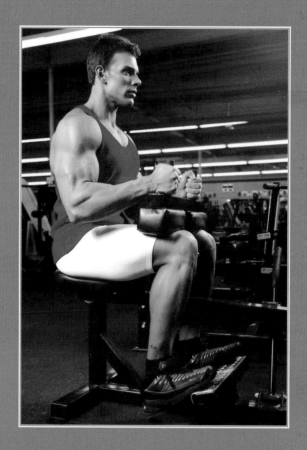

Seated
Calf Raise—
Machine

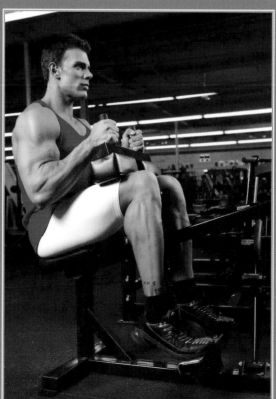

CALVES   EXERCISES

Seated Calf Raise—Machine

Sit up straight on the machine, and slide your knees under the kneepads. Place the balls of your feet flat on the footplate, lifting the kneepads up off the rest and to the starting position. Remove the rest. Inhale as you press up from your toes, slowly lifting your heels as high as you can above the level of the footplate. Then exhale as you slowly lower your heels down and as far below the footplate as you can.

Perfect form: Your ankles should be directly below your knees so that your lower legs point straight down throughout the motion.

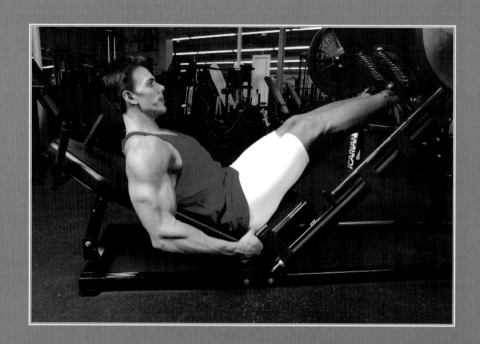

Toe Raise—
Machine

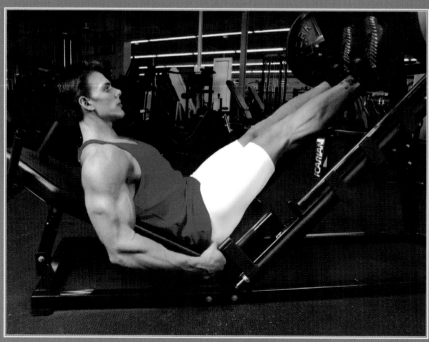

CALVES   EXERCISES

Toe Raise—Machine

Sit in a leg-press machine, and plant your feet on the footplate. Extend your legs without locking your knees, pressing the footplate up off its rests. Disengage the rests, and move your left foot down to the lower edge of the plate so that the weight rests on your toes. Remove your right foot from the plate and rest it on the ground. Inhale as you slowly extend your left foot, pressing the plate upward with your toes. Then exhale as you lower the plate back down with your toes. Complete your reps, switch feet, and perform the exercise with your right foot.

Perfect form: Keep your knees slightly bent, and lift only with your calves. Don't press from your thighs.

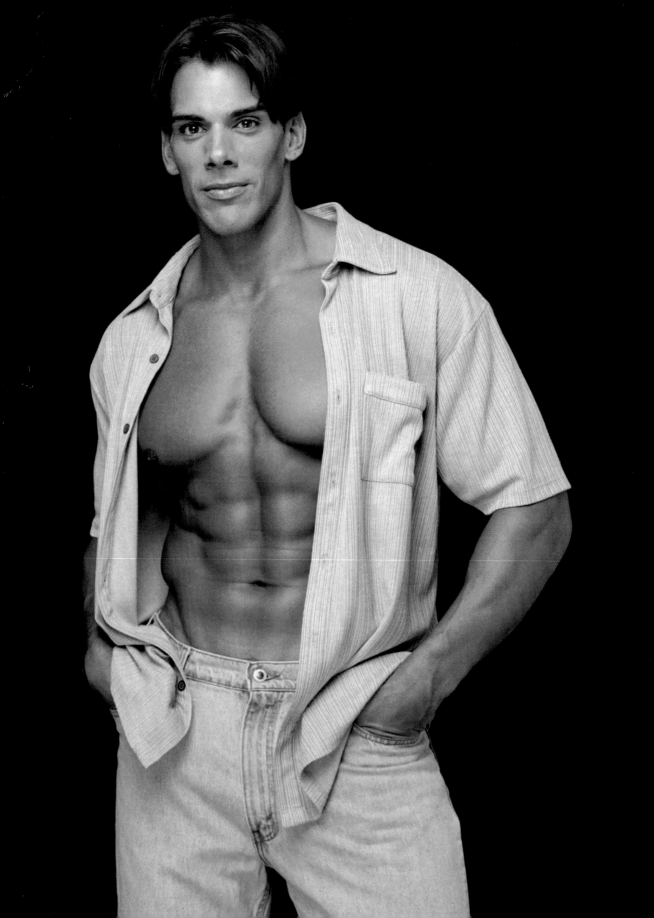

About the Author

To distill **Frank Sepe** in brief isn't as easy as one may think. Sure, as one of the planet's most formidable bodybuilders and physique models of all time, Frank has graced hundreds of magazine covers, romance-book jackets, and fitness encyclopedias; and he's been the subject of some 500 fan Websites. But this isn't nearly the full picture . . . not by a long shot.

Frank is also a highly respected fitness expert who's a contributing editor and monthly columnist for leading magazines *(MuscleMag International, American Health and Fitness)*; a consultant/fitness source for TV programs such as *Inside Edition* and *Hard Copy,* as well as for top women's Websites and magazines (Oxygen, *Cosmopolitan)*; and a working actor *(The Devil and Daniel Webster, Carlito's Way)* who's made frequent TV appearances *(Live with Regis and Kelly,* VH1, *The Howard Stern Show, Late Night with Conan O'Brien)*. He also maintains private personal-training clients (including celebrities and professional athletes) and is a spokesperson for fitness giant MET-Rx—all while promoting accredited physique and fitness shows throughout the U.S.

To contact Frank, please e-mail: **mail@franksepe.com**.

We hope you enjoyed this Hay House book.
If you would like to receive a free catalog featuring additional
Hay House books and products, or if you would like information
about the Hay Foundation, please contact:

Hay House, Inc.
P.O. Box 5100
Carlsbad, CA 92018-5100

(760) 431-7695 or **(800) 654-5126**
(760) 431-6948 (fax) or **(800) 650-5115 (fax)**
www.hayhouse.com

Published and distributed in Australia by:
Hay House Australia, Ltd. • 18/36 Ralph St. • Alexandria NSW 2015 •
Phone: 612-9669-4299 • *Fax:* 612-9669-4144 • www.hayhouse.com.au

Published and Distributed in the United Kingdom by:
Hay House UK, Ltd. • Unit 202, Canalot Studios •
222 Kensal Rd., London W10 5BN • *Phone:* 44-20-8962-1230 •
*Fax:*44-020-8962-1239 • www.hayhouse.co.uk

Published and Distributed in the Republic of South Africa by:
Hay House SA (Pty), Ltd., P.O. Box 990, Witkoppen 2068 •
Phone/Fax: 2711-7012233 • orders@psdprom.co.za

Distributed in Canada by:
Raincoast • 9050 Shaughnessy St., Vancouver, B.C. V6P 6E5 •
Phone: (604) 323-7100 • *Fax:* (604) 323-2600